LIVE IN KNOWLEDGE

LIVE IN KNOWLEDGE

AFTER THE PANDEMIC

Narrator Sri Baheti

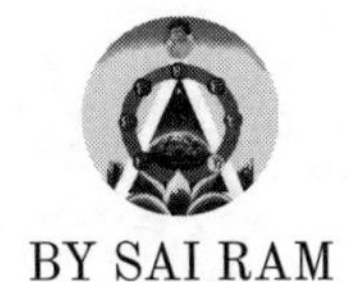

BY SAI RAM

Contents

First Printing, 2020

Introduction

Human beings are a vibrant species in this universe. Many members of this vibrant species indulge in the quest for the unknown in their life time.

This quest drives various researches and various theories get established. Many of these theories are denied by future scientists and researchers. The reason is that there is no concrete evidence for these theories.

Many research scientists, over various centuries, have kept on imagining and applying it practically to improve the quality of human life. This was done according to Hinduism by Rishis and Munis, who were essentially the scientists of those eras. Since these individuals were always withdrawn within themselves, the theories they established were based on logics developed internally in the mind and came to Hinduism as Vedas, puranas, and Upanishads, which described the ways to live through yoga, ayurveda, astrology and many such sciences.

The objective of all these researches was to enrich the human life with happiness and freedom from disease. Some of the rishis also talked about attaining immortality and various powers which could be obtained by human beings. This knowledge of powers and how to obtain them by various humans of not so noble nature created a divide between noble and knowledgeable humans called devas on one side, and the not so noble humans called demons or asuras on the other. In present times, also we have some very noble people who are a happier lot and a not so noble people, who are unhappier comparatively. The stories say that the happier people live in

heaven and the unhappier ones live in hell, while still living in this world

Since both of these human qualities have different powers, different ways to live, and different objectives, there used to be quarrels and wars between them. All the Hindu scriptures have narrated many such wars which have been fought between devas and asuras/demons and many results have been narrated.

Many Godly personalities were involved in this war to triumph over evil personalities and that is the essence of Hinduism to make us a good human being rather than getting lost into many such demonic qualities which we are all susceptible to.

All the religions talk about becoming better human beings. But, other than in Hinduism, where many such personalities have been named, all other religions have been centered around one personality. That is the difference between religions as such. Otherwise all religions want us to become better human beings.

Many knowledgeable people have tried to link science and religion. This book has also attempted to do the same besides delving into the ways and means to this knowledge to enrich the quality of life that a human being enjoys on this earth.

The present day science is more directed towards achievements. So you need a fulfilled life with achievements in some form or the other. However achievements can also be divided into noble achievements and worldly achievements, which may not be so noble. Many books, including management science books, have been written for the worldly achievements. But in Hindu scriptures they say, "if you acquire the knowledge then you will surely attain all the four legs of achievements that is dharma (duty), artha (money), kama

(desires), and moksha (liberation). Would it not be a better life if you live doing your duties, while also ensuring that you create happiness?

Similarly if such a man also has money in his life he enjoys life while fulfilling his desires and then when death nears he is so knowledgeable that after exhausting all his impressions he gets liberated from the sufferings of this world and dies a happy man. In other words, both this world and the world beyond, which is a liberated world, will be made available to such person. That is why an attempt is being made to give you the knowledge linked with science to let you know how you can get the advantage of both the worlds all the time. I strongly believe that it is important not to have undercurrents of doubts and anxiety. Each of us have characteristics and mental attitudes; so everyone judges things according to his own perspective and talks and argues in the light of his or her own nature. But there is one eternally right path, which with our own wisdom, own resolution and without getting effected by popular appraisal we should follow.

The good always provoke the bad into calumny; the bad always provoke the good into derision. This is the nature of the world. However truth certainly triumphs so we should do our rightful duty and not get affected.

This book also aims to help you to understand and then decide for yourself what your right path is for a healthier, happier, and longer life.

Hope the readers enjoy the small attempt made with a lot of affection to all the readers.

-

Acknowledgement

- *I must acknowledge the help in refining the book in its present shape to Shyam Nair who gave some wonderful touch to the book.*
- *I also acknowledge Guru Braja K. Parida in consciously making me understand some portions*
- *I acknowledge the contribution by Umakant Rana for his wonderful help in coordinating the making of this book.*

Disclaimer

The narrator, publisher, and anyone else does not claim any responsibility of the contents of this book as true and therefore the book can be essentially considered as a work of fiction and any resemblance to any person may be pure coincidental and not intentional.

-

1

Searching for Answers!

The evening of January 5th, 2020, was as fine as any that winter. I was relaxing at home in Reading, MA, with my wife, Stella, and daughter, Ruth. The setting sun formed a perfect backdrop as I sat on my favorite chair, partly reminiscing about the recently concluded year-end celebrations and partly contemplating on what the New Year would have in store for me and my business. By contemplating, I do not mean in a pensive sort of way, for the signs were all very good – the economy was on the upswing, unemployment numbers were at their lowest in quite some time, and the stock market was booming, creating wealth for investors. I was simply looking forward to a wonderful new year of wealth and happiness.

Ruth, I knew, was in the backyard playing with the snow that had not yet melted with the change of the year. I could hear Stella pottering about in the kitchen, busily humming to

herself. Unbidden, the famous lines from Robert Browning's poem came to my mind:-

The year's at the spring,
And day's at the morn;
Morning's at seven;
The hill-side's dew-pearl'd;
The lark's on the wing;
The snail's on the thorn;
God's in His heaven –
All's right with the world!

One could, of course, argue that the poem hadn't got several things right. Spring was a couple of months away and morning, as delightful as it promised to be, was still separated from me by a hopefully restful night. The lark and the snail concerned me not. But God certainly seemed to be perfectly in control, in heaven, and all seemed indeed to be right with the world.

I inhaled the delicious aroma that was floating in from the kitchen and rose from my chair in anticipation of a good meal. As was my habit during dinner, I switched on my regular news channel. Somehow, even the most appetizing of meals always felt incomplete to me without my daily dose of dinner-time news. The news was only a kind of white noise that I liked to have in the background, even as my family continued to indulge in dinner-time conversations. In the first couple of months of our marriage, Stella had seemed bothered by my habit, but she had gotten used to it. I guess it was

simply one of those many, mildly irritating things that I had picked up from my father.

Like I said, the news never really interfered with my family's dinner conversations. So, I only heard the anchor talking about this new virus that had surfaced in China in the passing. The anchor did not seem unusually perturbed by the information that she was passing on to her viewers. I was only partly paying attention to her because my mind had already raced ahead to thinking about getting back to work after my year-end holidays the next day. My thoughts were already focusing on the targets that I was planning to set for myself and my team for the New Year. And that probably explains why this bit of news bypassed my conscious mind to reside in some unexplored alley of my subconscious. After dinner, I continued to mindlessly surf channels for a while and then retired to bed, hoping to rise early and fresh the next morning to take on the world.

Three days later, with the weekend looming, the only thing on my mind was the get together that we had planned with the Harrisons, Brenda and James. James and I went back a long way, right from the time that we had gone to college together.

On Friday evening, I went out to dinner with a couple of buddies to a restaurant in Boston. There, in the middle of a gripping game between the Cavaliers and the Pistons, I spotted an insignificant ticker about the virus situation in Wuhan, China. I may also have overheard some folks on the table across from us talking about it. But, I wasn't going to let something that was happening halfway across the globe spoil

my appetite, and pushed the news once more to the back of my mind.

After coming home, I did check to see if there was anything serious brewing. But all the news anchors were falling over one another to assure the viewers that the US had nothing to worry about and that China was taking control of the virus.

It was only on January 21st, when the same anchors started talking about how the virus had made its way to South Korea, thanks to just one person who had travelled to Seoul from China, that the alarm bells started ringing. The anchors continued to hold on to their "the-US-has-nothing-to-worry-about" attitude. That, coupled with the fact that China was so far away and that we had some of the best scientists in the world, lulled me into silencing those alarm bells one more time. In that famous, resilient way of all Americans, I continued to be absorbed in my work and matters at home as usual. In my defense, I must let you know that I was planning a business trip to Florida in early February, and that, possibly also helped me to roast my worries on the backburner. Sunny Florida would be such a welcome relief from the bitter cold of Boston, I thought, looking forward to a round of golf with some potential business partners.

By January 30th, the situation had changed dramatically and the alarm bells were ringing louder than ever. The virus now had a name – COVID 19. This is a significant event. You usually don't bother naming something until it has assumed noteworthy proportions. The World Health Organization certainly seemed to think that this virus, one of many of the Corona family, was now a significant enough threat to

the world at large to deserve a name of its own. It had now reached Japan, was rising significantly in numbers in South Korea, and killing substantial numbers in Wuhan.

However, like every cloud, this one had a silver lining, too. Most of those who had been infected had been in direct contact with people who had acquired the virus in Wuhan. There was no local transmission in South Korea or Japan. While I was encouraged by this fact, I continued to sense a growing uneasiness in the back of my mind where I had left my worries to barbeque. 'What would happen', I wondered, 'were someone infected in Wuhan to travel to the US. After all, wasn't it just a matter of time before such an event did actually happen?'

It didn't take long for my question to be answered. Apparently, a person infected with the virus had travelled from China to the US on January 20th. The threat was now very real and the government was taking it rather seriously and had set up a taskforce to deal with it.

That night, at dinner, I voiced my concerns to Stella. She smiled indulgently and teasingly called me a "worrier". But, it was clear that she could see that my "worrying" was not without reason. But that was how she was. Ever the practical one, she would soak in my worries like a sponge and inevitably come up with a solid solution.

Not surprisingly, it didn't take her long to come up with something this time as well.

'John', she said, 'do you remember Anand guruji?'

I was surprised that Stella had asked. There were two reasons for this. For one, no one who had met Anand guruji

even once in life was ever likely to forget him. For another, I had been thinking about him quite a bit that day.

'Of course', I replied, 'why do you ask?'

'Remember what he had said about the world encountering a serious situation sometime in March, this year?'

My mind raced to a time about five months prior to the present. Stella, Ruth, and I had been to India on a holiday in August 2019. Among the many wonderful people we had met there was this guru, named Anand. One particular conversation that I had with guruji, to which Stella was referring, was now playing clearly in my mind. He had indeed told us that the world would encounter a very serious situation in or around March 2020.

'Why don't we call guruji and ask him about his thoughts on the current situation?' Stella asked. Apart from being the practical one, she was also the more spontaneous one in the marriage. Once a solid idea, at least according to her, took root in her mind, then she'd move heaven and earth to see to it that it was accomplished. Going to India in the middle of a stressful third quarter had been an idea that had sprung in that stubborn mind as well.

My watch showed that it was nearly 10 in the night. I quickly calculated that it would be around a half past seven in the morning in India. I knew that guruji would have been up and about since four in the morning. He had said that the pre-dawn hours were particularly auspicious. He had even referred to that particular time by a name, which I could not now remember.

Assuring myself that I had nothing to lose, I dialed his number. His voice, when he answered the phone, was as calm

as I always remembered it. Indian gurus, especially the more articulate ones such as Anand guruji, are very busy people. So, I was surprised to find that he not only remembered me, but also Stella and Ruth and politely enquired after them. After the initial exchange of pleasantries, I cut to the chase. 'Guruji', I asked, 'do you remember the conversation we had where you told me that the world would see some difficult times in March 2020?'

'Yes, I do.'

'Were you, by any chance, speaking of the virus that's now threatening to spread across the world?'

I could almost see the calm smile that had so often lit up guruji's face during our conversations. 'You sound worried. Why worry when whatever has to happen will happen anyway.'

'Guruji, why is this happening?' asked Stella, unable to keep herself out of the conversation, 'How long will this last? Is there any way that we could protect ourselves?'

'Let me ask you a question', said guruji, in reply, 'are you looking only at protecting yourselves from this virus or would you be interested in knowing how to lead a happy and healthy life for as long as you are in this world?'

'Well, it would be nice to be healthy and happy always, guruji, but the fact is that the virus is the immediate threat.'

'Ok, let's suppose that I tell you how to deal with this virus now. But what if there was another virus that threatened to shake the world to its very foundations a couple of years down the line? Would you then seek a remedy for that virus, too?'

'Hmm…' replied Stella, beginning to realize the wisdom of guruji's words.

'Trying to deal with this one virus is like trying to treat the symptoms of a disease. You may be successful in dealing with it, for now. But symptoms lie low for a while and then resurface in a more malignant form. But, if you choose to focus on leading a happy and healthy life, you'd be actually dealing with the underlying disease itself. Needless to say, if you treat the disease, the symptoms will die out as well.'

'But', continued guruji, 'if you really want to understand what it means to be happy and healthy, then you will have to understand the science behind it. As a bonus, you will also learn how to tide past the present crisis as well. But, this knowledge, which is a part of Indian culture, will only come to you if you have a serious desire to learn it. Knowledge comes only to those that seek it with all their heart.'

Both Stella and I were deeply intrigued. 'If there was science involved', I reasoned, 'I may be actually able to connect with it.' I heard myself say, 'We are ready, guruji.' There was a twinkle of merriment in guruji's voice, when he replied, 'Oh! Are you? I am glad to know that you think so. Let me warn you that there is no mantra that I can give you. If you are a serious seeker, you must be prepared to begin at the very beginning and understand what life is. We must seek answers to questions like why we are born and what our purpose in life is. We must understand what the different aspects of life are, and then, perhaps, we will learn how we may emerge out of the present crisis, unscathed. There are no shortcuts. So, my friends please commit to this journey only if you are in it for the long haul!'

'Could there really be a purpose for our birth?' I thought. The look on Stella's face told me that she was also thinking on the same lines. Suddenly, I realized that I really wanted to know the answers to these questions. 'Guruji, I really want to know the answers to these questions', I heard myself saying, 'and I'm ready to begin at the beginning and spend what time is required.'

'Think of it as an investment, John', replied guruji soothingly. 'I know you like and understand that word very well. Trust me when I say that it's a wise investment. But, like all other good investments, it pays the best returns only if you stay invested in it for as long as is required. Let's start tomorrow at 10 PM EST on Skype. Each session will be two hours long, and we'll need an entire week to talk about all the things that you'd need to know.'

Somewhere in the back of my mind was the thought, 'Hey! Don't I have a say in this? Shouldn't guruji at least be checking with me if the time was convenient to me?' Over the course of the following week, I was to learn that the imparting of knowledge in the traditional Indian way was significantly different from how it was done in the western world. The guru, or the source of knowledge, was a revered figure and humility and compliance was the hallmark of a student, the seeker of knowledge. For the moment, I pushed my thoughts away and agreed to set up the call as instructed by guruji.

Little was I to know, then, that I was about to embark on the most intriguing journey of my life with the call the next day.

2

Game of Energy!

Sometimes we went out bowling with our friends, Brenda and James Harrison. This was usually followed by dinner at a favorite restaurant. But we were a little distracted that day as the impending discussion with guruji that was scheduled for after dinner was looming in our minds. The Harrisons must have noticed that we were preoccupied, but didn't say anything about it. During dinner, possibly just to initiate a discussion to end the unusual awkwardness that had descended between us friends, I asked James if he had ever reflected on why humans are born.

'What a silly thing to ask, John!' exclaimed James, 'If the male and female energies interact then we are born and that is a very normal answer.' Stella and I nodded in agreement. James was right. That was the only "normal" answer, or, at least the only one that we were aware of. I told the Harrisons about our interactions with guruji and said, 'If the answer was as simple as that, would guruji have asked us this question?'

Ruth, not wanting to be left out of the conversation, piped in, 'The doctors at the hospital were the reason for my birth.

So that should be the answer.' We all laughed at her innocence and agreed that yes that was possibly the smartest answer.

Brenda asked, 'But Bible says that we are all born out of sin. So is lovemaking sin?'

"What nonsense!" exclaimed James?

We agreed that it would be wiser to wait to hear what Guruji had to say. We promised the Harrisons that we'd let them know exactly what guruji thought about the subject. We finished dinner and hurried home to begin our session with guruji.

'What is your concept of God?' With this question, guruji launched our ship down the river of knowledge.

'Wow!' I thought, 'straight to "the" point. Not beating around the bush, are we? Wouldn't that be a question we might be able to answer after we have completed our course?'

I reflected upon this question that guruji had posed. What did I think of God? Did I actually ever really think of God? Was God in my thoughts as often as Stella or Ruth were? I thought of God when I went to church on Sundays. God was on my mind when the stock markets were swinging wildly, sending my heart racing like an F1 race car. God did find a place in my thoughts when something unexpectedly worrying had happened at work or at home. Other than that, I didn't really have a concept of God.

As if guessing my thoughts, guruji asked, 'Do you think that's a tough question? Please understand that questions are never tough. Also be aware that your answer to the same question will change as your knowledge increases. So don't even for a moment think that you answer is insignificant.

It is simply a reflection of what you know at the moment when the question was asked. All I am asking is, what, with the knowledge you have at present, do you understand about God?'

"I'm just not sure that I have a concept of God, really', I said, measuring my words carefully. 'I know that I think of God at times. I know I also sometimes blame God for misfortunes in my life. I have sometimes felt that there was a helping hand when I needed it the most, but the same hand was conspicuous by its absence at other, equally desperate times. I have never actively searched for God, so I have never found him. How did man find God, anyway?"

Guruji replied, "Necessity, John! Necessity is the mother of invention. It is true that human beings, over a period of time, have realized that any amount of external achievement would not bring lasting happiness if there was an absence of inner satisfaction. However, before this realization, they feared the various forces of nature. There was a time when mankind feared the wrath of nature, be it in the form of rains, floods, or earthquakes. They were utterly incapable of comprehending the incredible display of force that nature sometimes put up for them. It was easier for them to think of these phenomena as the wrath of some all-pervading entity called God, whose displeasure they had somehow incurred. There was no way for our early ancestors to attribute a scientific basis to these natural phenomena that a fourth-grader could possibly explain today. Think about it, can we honestly say that we have overcome our fear of the unknown entirely even today? Think about your own fear of Covid-19. Don't you fear it because you are unable to comprehend it? Uncer-

tainty and the terrible questions that life poses is what makes people want to try and understand god. When you are happy, you are aware of the reason for your emotion. You do not think of god, then, because no explanation is needed for your emotion. But if you are sad and you cannot fathom why that feeling has taken root in your heart, you seek god, to ask why. When you don't know, you must seek. Admitting your ignorance and seeking answers is a powerful tool that the ancient wise men of India used to seek god. In that process, they unearthed a vast treasure of knowledge that is impossible to fathom. This conversation of ours also has its origins in your inner desire to understand god and creation.'

Stella stepped into the conversation. 'Guruji, we are Christians. To us Jesus Christ is god.'

Guruji said, "Indeed, he is a godly figure because of his godly qualities. So, why do some people who are born on earth have these godly qualities? Why does history, sometimes passed down as mythology, remember such people who are endowed with divine qualities thousands of years after they have passed from this world? To understand that, you must understand that behind these godly qualities is a science that you must become aware of.'

I may have looked skeptical. Even Stella, who was good at maintaining a deadpan expression when the situation demanded it, was raising an eyebrow.

Guruji acknowledged this, and said, 'Sounds weird doesn't it? Science seeks logic and proof, which are apparently completely absent in the concept of god. To many people, god and science are therefore mutually exclusive. Or, are they? I will now attempt to explain what I had meant when I said that

there was a science behind this concept of god. Science says that the godly qualities or positive energy in human beings is a part of the total energy in the universe. All human beings are made out of atoms. In their ionic states, these atoms can either have an excess number of protons in their nuclei or extra electrons in their orbits. And the atoms are all along vibrating. A combination of these vibrating atoms is what we see as the human body.

Ever since Albert Einstein gave the world the famous equation $E = MC^2$, that we have all understood, or at least remember from school, even the western world acknowledges that all of life is energy. It means that the energy contained in a body is equivalent to mass multiplied by the speed of light squared. But what does it really mean? It means that all of life — everything that exists – the atom and molecule, every blade of grass, every speck of dust, and the ray of the sun — is made up of energy. And of course, it means that we are energy, too…full of atoms vibrating inside us.'

Guruji paused to see if we had absorbed all that he had said. 'Do you agree now that the creation of the universe is due to energy?'

'I agree, guruji', I said, 'but what has this to do with god?'

'Patience, John', said guruji, with a smile. 'Let us think of an indescribable, infinite energy cloud consisting of trillions of atoms with electrons, filled with electronic charge. Let's call this cloud God. This kind of energy cannot be seen or experienced, much like our concept of God. Now, suppose that there has been an extra clouding of electrons in this huge mass. Would not the electrons at the extremities of this cloud slip out? It is like the subdivision of an atom where you

have loose electrons spilling out leaving the atom positively charged.'

'Hmm...' said Stella, 'much like when the water content in a rain cloud exceeds a certain percentage, the water falls to the Earth as rain!'

'Exactly!' said guruji, 'the electrons and the energy particles which are at the extreme ends do try to get detached from the huge mass in the manner that I just described and that is the start of energy.'

I was struck by this powerful visualization. God as energy was such a fantastic thought.

Guruji continued, 'When the electrons get detached, a sound is created. This is easy to visualize. Even a simple phenomenon like the tearing of a paper creates a sound. So, the sound energy becomes the first energy when the energy particles divide or separate. The sound energy is essentially a propagation taking place due to the harmonic motion of the atoms. This "creation" of energy is known as "*Bramha*" in Hindu mythology. This universal sound is heard as "OM". Please imagine how this would sound in space where there is total vacuum! Wouldn't it sound like waterfall of electrons cascading down endlessly? You can actually experience this OHHHHHM sound flowing also within your body. All you need to do is plug your ears with your fingers, close your eyes, and then concentrate. Please try it.'

I did as instructed. Sure enough, I heard the sound and it did sound like "OM".

'OM is the sound energy', said guruji, 'and it is considered the energy of creation. In the bible, doesn't John 1:1 speak of

god as the word and the Holy Ghost, the vibration, and as amen, the witness?'

Guruji sat quietly for a minute, letting all that had been said sink in.

'Now' continued guruji, 'please understand that we are talking about splitting or separating atoms and electrons in its outer orbit that are clinging together. When electrons are thrown out, a second form of energy, light, is also created. We know that light is essential for the process of photosynthesis in plants, and, as a corollary, for life in general on Earth. So, can we think of light as the "source of life"? This second form of energy, the 'life-giver' or 'savior', is called "Vishnu" in Hindu mythology.'

'When we are speaking of energy, we are speaking of a heavy electrical charge at probably trillions of volts. Such a high charge would necessarily be accompanied by heat energy, wouldn't it? This heat energy, or fire, is the third energy and the cause of destruction in the universe. In Hindu mythology, this is described as "Mahesh". Every person or object is created or destroyed by using these three, eternal energies.'

'Nature operates as these energies to create, preserve, and destroy or dissolute. A wave that is created in an ocean is preserved for a moment before dissolving back into the vast ocean. Similarly, the life force creates all of us, preserves us for a while, and then we all dissolve back into it.

However these three energies all emanate from powerful trillions of volts of energy source, which we all can call as god.

Let me tell you a story, here. Let us presume that all these energies, Bramha, Vishnu, and Mahesh were actually humans

with the powers of the energies that they represent vested in them. Let's think of them as superheroes, much like your avenger movie characters. One day Brahma, Vishnu, and Mahesh were arguing as to who was the most powerful of them all. The argument was becoming more and more heated by the minute and no end was in sight. That's when a fourth person entered the scene. 'Ah!' said our superheroes, 'here comes one who shall judge who among us is the mightiest!' Saying thus, they reached out to the newcomer with their query. The newcomer decided to interview the candidates. 'You are the creator, you say', he said to Bramha, 'but what is it that you create?' Bramha, the wise replied loftily, 'Everything!' The man then turned to Vishnu and asked, 'What is it that you do?' 'I am the preserver,' came the reply. Mahesh, when his turn came, informed the man that his job was to destroy.

'Very important tasks, all three!' mused the man, 'but I must see these powers put to test for myself before I can crown one of you the mightiest.' Saying so, the man picked a straw and handed it to Bramha. 'Please create this straw for me this very instant, O venerable creator', he said. Whether within his three heads, Bramha considered this task below his dignity, we shall never know. However, being as true a contestant as there ever was, the venerable one focused on creating the straw. But try as he might, he was unable to create the straw instantly. This was no wonder, however, because even a thing as simple as a straw is created in accordance to the laws of nature. Even the creator cannot violate these laws and create anything instantly. With as much dignity as he

could muster, Bramha handed the humble piece of straw to the man.

It was now Vishnu's turn to show the true extent of his powers. The man turned to Vishnu and proffered the same straw to the preserver of the universe with the simple request, 'preserve this straw, O Vishnu.' Alas, this, too, was against the laws of nature. The sun was beating down mercilessly on the poor straw, drying it out, and nothing that Vishnu could do was enough to stop this from happening.

It was then Mahesh's turn to do his bit. 'Destroy this straw, O great destroyer', requested the man. Mahesh burned down the straw and looked around in triumph. However, the fair judge pointed to the ashes and said, 'you haven't destroyed it, after all.'

I was listening to guruji's story with rapt attention. 'Guruji, I asked, 'does this mean that there is a greater power than this Holy Trinity in Hinduism?'

'In Hinduism, we consider that there is a greater power that created the laws of nature. According to us, Purusha, the ultimate energy or god and prakriti, or nature, are intertwined. They can only create, preserve, or destroy according to the laws of nature. It is certain that they act through the three energies which are responsible for the functions allotted to them.'

'We find such laws in the entire universe. Have you ever wondered why the stars and planets continue in their respective orbits without colliding? This is also due to these laws, created by the universal law creator, who we name god. God is omnipresent, omniscient, and omnipotent.'

'But, guruji', I persisted, 'how did man find god?'

'When man shuts himself from the world and concentrates on discovering the intelligence behind the universal law by doing away with the consciousness of matter, then god reveals itself. That is how the ancient rishis of India, the earliest scientists of mankind, discovered a part of this intelligence. Are you surprised that I used the word scientist to refer to the rishis? If a scientist is someone that does research to discover something or delve deeper into a subject, then there is no more apt term than "scientist" to refer to a rishi, in my opinion. The ancient rishis were always undertaking research to know the creator and its laws.'

The idea of a large mass of electrons and energy produced by the separation of these electrons got me thinking. 'Guruji', I ventured, 'why does this remind me of the Big Bang Theory?'

'Excellent observation!' That's simply because the Big Bang Theory agrees with this concept entirely. Remember that it started with a "bang", or a sound, caused by the separation of some mass from the larger body of mass. The light and heat energies that followed became the sustainer and destroyer respectively of life. Initially when everything was a vacuum and when there was complete darkness in the universe, these three energies by themselves could not create life. However, the continuous burning created a matter mass which also was burning initially. Inert gases existed, but could not create life by themselves. The foundation of life was laid when the inert gases, especially helium, broke down to form hydrogen, due to the extreme, unimaginably high temperature of the fire energy. This hydrogen, while burning, created carbon as the first matter. A burning fire creates ash, doesn't

it? That's essentially what happened here as well. The carbon-hydrogen combination, often known as the "CH combination", is the basis of creation of all matter in the universe.'

As always, guruji paused, giving us a minute to absorb all that we had heard.

'The Hindu mythology also talks about "Saptrishis." In Sanskrit, "Sapt" means seven. Mythology speaks of these seven great rishis as demigods because they remained within themselves and never reacted with anything or anybody. This is simply an allegory for the seven inert gases, helium, neon, argon, krypton, xenon, radon, and flerovium that we know of in modern science. According to mythology, these Rishis were asked to continue the process of creation by Bramha, the primeval sound energy. However, they failed to do so by themselves. It was then that these inert gases were broken down to create life. Hydrogen and carbon combined to create different life forms. Did you know that there are allegorical references to this in Christianity?'

'Do you mean the story of Adam and Eve in the Book of Genesis, guruji?' ventured Stella.

'Absolutely!' exclaimed guruji, sounding rather pleased. 'In Hindu mythology, we have the story of Manu and Sathrupa. Two entities coming together and life bursting forth from their union!'

'Good lord!' I exclaimed, as the science or logic behind the explanation struck me. The Big Bang Theory itself was known to almost everybody who had attended High School. But how many had understood it in this way? Could an ancient civilization have explored the depths of this theory and

come out with a logical explanation? From what I had heard thus far, it certainly seemed to have been the case.

'For the present, let us concentrate on our sun and solar system and what happened when the matter started cooling down. On Earth, the cooling matter created magnetic fields. Some of the inert gases were electrified and broken down giving their saturated electrons and that is how other gases including oxygen was created. This newly evolved gas combined with hydrogen, creating water, laying the foundations of life as we know it today. As most of us know today, it is widely accepted that life forms originated in the ocean and then evolved into the other earthly life forms.'

It looked to me like we were venturing into the deeper realms of the science of evolution. Was it connected in some way to the evolution of the virus that had prompted this entire discussion?

'But guruji, what about us humans? How were we created?'

3

The Science of Human Creation!

Next day, I asked, 'Guruji is there any parallel to how the virus has been created and how we, humans, have been created?' Guruji smiled, 'John, you surely know that the reproduction in viruses is not the same as in us, humans. But yes they are also born out of Mother Nature and function as per the laws of nature, exactly like all of us. It is for us to understand and decipher the laws of nature and that is true not only in creation but in living and destruction as well. The goal of life is to make sure that every aspect of our lives follows the laws of nature so as that we remain happy and trouble free. Guruji said 'Therefore in every aspect of life if we understand and follow the law of nature we will remain happy. So let me first tell you how we humans evolved. If we were to put it simply, purely aquatic life graduated to amphibious life, which in time graduated to land animals. There was a transitory half animal-half human form, which then graduated to the human form as we know it today."

'Let's for the moment leave this "evolutionary" concept aside and focus on the creation of a human life. Medical science tells us that this is achieved when a sperm enters an egg without breaking it. The sperm is an alkaline medium and the egg is an acidic substance. High School science tells us that the combination of an acid and an alkali results in an exothermic reaction. Simply put, heat is generated within the egg when the alkaline sperm combines with the acidic egg. This heat is not distributed evenly within the egg. There are different temperature zones. This difference of temperature in different zones creates an electric current within the egg.

This electric current forces the excretion of a chemical fine print of the sperm and the egg. The pineal glands secrete the first substance around the 49th day of the conception, and this is the beginning of life. By life, we mean movement and this is the first movement caused by the continuous temperature difference in different zones. The secretion then moves to the pituitary gland and subsequently to the thyroid gland. By the time it moves to the heart, a substantial electromagnetic field is formed. The secretion then further goes down to create the solar plexus – the reproductive gland associated with the Swadhisthan chakra and the adrenal gland associated with the Mooladhar chakra. According to science, the sulfur and mercury in the sperm and the egg combine to create mercuric sulfide and that first creates the chemical compound known as rasa in the body. Thereafter, blood, muscle, fat, bone, bone marrow, and reproductive organs are progressively created and ojas, which is the temperature difference current, starts flowing in the body.

These are essentially the seven chakras of the body as de-

scribed in Hinduism. Life really starts from the penile gland and ends at the adrenal gland. The excess of adrenal secretion is the natural cause of death. The heat energy created is pushed down and settles in the lower-most area of the human body – the reproductive glands. The temperature difference between the zones of the reproductive glands and the pineal glands creates an electric current which essentially drives the heart. When the temperature difference between the two zones becomes zero, the electric current is stopped and life ends. Essentially, it is the temperature in the body which is life. How do we keep this heat energy alive? By eating, or adding fuel to this fire. The alkaline and acidic chemicals are stored at different places in the body and are secreted separately though they do combine to create different compounds of chemicals. The alkaline content remains with the bones and the acidic content more with the enzymes in the liver. Thus the body constitutes a balanced pH ratio. This is like imagining a dry cell battery running with zinc and sulfuric acid thereby releasing the electrical energy required to drive any of our gadgets. Therefore whatever we eat, the excess of acid or alkali gets deposited in the organ warehouse in excess of chemical reaction required to maintain the temperature. During this chemical reaction residue or ash is also formed as if there is a fire burning. If this is not eliminated properly along with the water content in the body, it becomes mucus and gets deposited in various organs giving rise to various diseases.'

'Are these deposits the cause of all diseases?' I asked.

Guruji casually replied, 'It seems to me that you are still focused on diseases. You could choose to know only about

diseases or partake in this universal knowledge that I'm trying to impart. But, before you make a choice, let me caution you that without knowing what needs to be known, you will not be able to understand how to prevent diseases or how to cure them. The many secretions in our body are dependent on our life style and thought processes. If you choose not to understand these basics, the way forward may be difficult. So, choose what you will.'

'Guruji', said Stella, looking at me sharply, 'we are here for the knowledge. Please go on.'

Guruji smiled and said that undoubtedly pure knowledge becomes boring to hear and assimilate but once we know it, this becomes our biggest gain of life and continued, 'mucus deposits are acidic in nature and get stuck to the various organs of the body and creates diseases. Death occurs when the alkaline substances in the body are over or consumed by the acidic substances, thus tilting the pH balance to the acidic side." So, in short, we can say that lifestyle is responsible for excess depletion of alkaline substance in our body and thus shortening our life cycle.'

"How long is a human body designed to survive for, guruji?' I asked.

Guruji said, 'well, normally the body is designed to live for a hundred and twenty years. But, we are all unable to make it that far because of our lifestyles and environmental reasons. So before you know about diseases, your emphasis should be to know the lifestyle that will help you to reduce diseases in the body. Our lifestyle should be essentially as close to the laws of nature as possible.

I asked, 'Guruji is it not true that the laws of nature keep

law did not discriminate whether the crime was committed knowingly or unknowingly.'

I pondered over this story a bit.

Guruji continued, 'Here's another story for you to reflect upon. In the Indian film industry, there were two friends. Let's call them Sid and Jeet. Jeet had written a story, which he was hoping to share with some producers to make into a film. But, his friend, Sid, stole the story from him and sold it off as his own. He made quite a bit of money on that account. Needless to say, that was the end of that friendship. Sid, who was now a rich man, disregarded his old friend. Things continued on that note for quite some time. Many years later the same Sid, who was now accustomed to hobnobbing with rich and famous producers, was gifted a heritage painting by one of them. Before he knew it, he was charged with the theft of the painting by the government. It is important to understand that Sid had not actually stolen the painting. He merely happened to have it in his possession and that was a crime in itself.'

'But, guruji,' Stella asked, 'how can we be sure that Sid was paying for what he had done to Jeet?'

Guruji smiled. 'You are right, Stella', he said, 'we cannot always be sure about what crime are we being punished for. But, in this case, there is one small, rather ironical twist. The officer who was investigating the case happened to be none other than Jeet's son.'

Stella and I looked at each other. Guruji noticed and smiled. 'Sounds like stuff from movies, doesn't it? But aren't movies a reflection of life? I'm not saying that the effect always comes tagged with an identifier of the cause. All I'm say-

ing is that every cause will have an effect, whether delivered instantly or at its own time. Therefore, we must understand that our actions have their effects. We may face these effects within the same life time or sometimes even in our future births. This action is called karma.'

Guruji looked at his watch. 'We have had a fairly good session today. Tomorrow, we'll talk about karma and why we are born? Is chemical reaction the only reason for our birth or is there something more to it than just that.'

Stella asked me 'How is it possible to condense the conversation and let the Harrisons know?'

I replied, 'unless we record it and they are willing to spend time listening to the recording, whatever we say will not be convincing enough.'

'That sounds like a good idea', said Stella, 'It may also be of some help to others who like such discussions. But we have to take Guruji's permission for that.'

'Let's ask him.'

4

Your Birth and Karma!

I went to work the next day, as usual, but my mind was occupied with the talk that we had with guruji the evening before. I was still trying to wrap my head around a lot of things that we had talked about. I had never thought that there could be a scientific explanation for god. If there was an explanation, how could someone continue to be an atheist? Even being agnostic did not seem very cool anymore because it simply felt like sitting on the fence because you are too afraid to accept the explanation that guruji had provided. Did Hinduism really believe in these precepts? Did all Hindus believe in these precepts? I had many friends, who were practicing Hindus. I was starting to view them in a different light now.

And this whole business of karma, birth, and rebirth that guruji was promising to unfold today seemed too enticing a prospect. I could not wait to get my day over with so that I could go home and our session could begin.

Stella called me around midday as was her usual practice.

But she wasn't her usual breezy self. She seemed to be preoccupied, as if deeply contemplating something.

'John', she asked, 'are we all just bodies made of energy? So why does a particular collection of energy called John or Ruth matter to me so much?'

'Maybe there's more to it than what has been revealed so far to us. Perhaps, guruji is waiting for the right time to tell us about it', I offered in reply.

Stella sighed. 'I can't wait to learn more, John! This is all so confounding and intriguing at the same time!'

I couldn't agree with her more. Guruji had said that god is energy and we are part of that energy. Is that what was said in Genesis 1:27 - So God **created man** in his own image, in the **image of God** he **created** him? If we were just packets of energy, why were we on earth? What was the purpose of our birth? I was glad that guruji was going to address this question in our discussion today.

Before the call started I asked Guruji 'can we record our conversation for the benefit of others who may also want to share the knowledge that we get from you?'

Guruji said, 'Well, this knowledge was available with me last year also, when you both met me, but at that time I never volunteered to give any information about this knowledge or answers on normal questions which a human mind may ask. If humans want to go deeper than the surface, then there is a law of nature that one who wants this knowledge and want to seek it will get it somehow or other. The universal energies are attracted in that manner and therefore unless some people are ready and hungry for this, the value of what you

are about to hear will be lost on them. My advice thus is not to record it.'

'Have you ever thought why you were born as John Smith and not as President Eisenhower?'

I wondered why guruji had chosen Eisenhower over other more recent presidents. I could think of several reasons why I was not born as Eisenhower. For one, Eisenhower was born in 1890, a good eighty-five years before I landed on this planet. But, had guruji asked why I wasn't born as President Obama, I still wouldn't have had an answer. So, this was probably a trick question, I thought.

Guruji was clearly not expecting an answer, for he continued. 'The chemical reactions involved in the births of human beings and animals are the same. Why, then, are we so different? Why do different people have different thought processes? Why is everybody not the same?'

'To be able to answer these questions, we must understand the concept of karma. I'm sure that you've heard of karma.'

Stella asked, 'Doesn't karma mean punishment, guruji? I've heard people say things like that's karma for your actions.'

'On the contrary, karma simply means action. All the karma, or our actions in our lifetime, leaves impressions on our subconscious mind as to what led us to that karma or to act the way we did? Was that karma guided by lust? Was it done in anger? Was it done because of greed? Was it done because of attachment? Was it done out of pride? Was it done because of jealousy?'

'The impressions made by our karma on our subconscious mind remain as unfulfilled desires or lessons to be learned

in a future life. We are reborn or reincarnated in this world to fulfill those unfulfilled desires or to learn those unlearned lessons. So, our present birth is also a rebirth to fulfill some unfulfilled desires of our previous birth. So what should we do to avoid rebirth or reincarnation?'

'Leave no desires unfulfilled?' I ventured, hopefully.

Guruji laughed. 'How many desires will you be able to fulfill in this lifetime, John? Is there an end to desires?'

In that, guruji was certainly correct. I remembered how I had swung from one desire to another throughout my life. I had wanted a good education then a good job, and then I had wanted to climb up the ladder. I had wanted a good house, then a great house, followed by a farmhouse on the outskirts of Boston for my weekend retreats. Certainly, desires were endless and there was no way that I could fulfill them in one life time.

Guruji continued. 'The idea is to let go of desires. If you are able to keep your subconscious mind clean and devoid of any desires, then you will not need to be reborn or reincarnated in this world.'

Stella, who was listening with rapt attention, asked, 'Guruji, does the unfulfilled desire of a previous birth play a role in determining the circumstances of our present birth?'

Guruji's eyes gleamed with pleasure. 'That's a great question, Stella. It is indeed the nature of the unfulfilled desires that decides the unique chemical compositions with which each one of us is born.'

Stella persisted with this particular line of questioning. It was clear that she was hooked on to the topic. 'But guruji,

how is the karma of our past life transmitted to our present life?'

'Images remain in ether when you die. Your habits and thoughts stay with this image. We do not become angels with wings and halos around your head and play the harp while floating about on clouds as some cartoon movies would have us believe. Instead, we come back with similar habits in another body Reincarnation is an undisputable fact. But, it is never with the same body, same set of friends, or even in the same place. This movie that is your present life is shelved the moment you die. But it comes back in a revamped form in some other incarnation.'

'To give effect to the karma we are born with some chemical compositions. Different explanations exist as to why different chemical combinations and compositions exist and how they are created by the universe. The most ecstatic one is the Science of Astrology which explains how the different planets affect the different elements on this earth at different times.'

'But, astrology is not a science', I blurted out, and received a sharp dig in the ribs from Stella for my outburst.

'Oh! Is it not? What if there was a scientific explanation for this as well?' asked guruji.

He continued. 'Do you agree that high tides in the ocean are caused by the relative angle and closeness of the moon to the earth? Do you agree that its gravitational pull could possibly cause the water in our body to change its velocity and move toward the outer extremes of the body? Since the water content in blood is very high, blood also tends to react in a similar manner. This affects the cells, which, in turn affects

the thought process. Does that sound like science, John? If the moon can affect human beings in the manner that I just described, then why can't the other planets?'

'Because they are further away', I argued, not willing to throw in the towel even at the cost of receiving another Stella elbow in my ribs.

'Good point! But do you agree that all objects in space exert a gravitational influence on all other objects, irrespective of the distance between them? Sir Isaac Newton surely believed so. This degree of influence is not only determined by the distance between the two objects but also by their respective masses.'

I nodded, meekly. After all, which student of science had not heard of the universal law of gravitation proposed by Newton?

'So, planets, no matter how distant they are from us, influence the beings on Earth. Saturn affects the iron and zinc elements of the body while Mars affects the copper element.'

'In this context, let's focus on why we find people of such varied natures around us. Different sets of chemical combinations, some in excesses and some in shortages, are present in different human bodies and therefore we see a variety of natures among human beings. Some of us are courageous and extroverted and others timid and introverted.'

'Therefore, we can see that body's actions are sometimes dependent on the kind of chemicals it has. Think of it this way – we all have different chemicals in our body and each of these chemicals is within a prescribed range. Let's take one such chemical, which for the purposes of our discussion we shall assume to be a chemical that makes someone angry by

nature. The concentration of this chemical may be toward the higher end of the acceptable range in Person A and closer to the lower end of the acceptable range in Person B. Clearly, Person A will be short tempered by nature, while Person B will be calm. We have also just seen how the planets have different effects on different chemicals. So, is it then difficult to see how the planets may affect the nature of a person? Therefore there is a link between the astrological planetary combination under which you were born and the makeup of your nature as per the proportion of different chemicals in your body.'

To a person who had always looked upon astrology as mere humbug with no basis in science, this was a total revelation. Somewhere within me rose the uncomfortable feeling that several of the notions that I had built up over the years on various subjects were going to come crashing down in the course of the week.

Guruji paused, gazing keenly at us with his intelligent eyes as if he could read the clash of ideas that he had unleashed within our minds. Then, he continued, 'I must also warn you that the astrological chemicals have only an impelling tendency to pull you in a particular direction as dictated by the nature of the chemicals. But, there is something that we call willpower, which is a force that is available within all of us to resist such tendencies. Willpower can help us to overcome the impelling tendencies of chemicals and prevent them from becoming compelling behaviors. To put it simply, you can overcome potentially negative tendencies caused by the chemical composition of your body by exercising the power of your will. Will power is very important tool that most of

us, unfortunately, do not have it in sufficient strength. So, the impelling tendencies of the chemicals become our compelling tendencies and we act accordingly and generate good or bad karmas.'

'So, guruji, is there a way for us to apply the power of our will to do good deeds only and forever resist bad deeds?' I asked.

'Yes, John, there is. We'll get to that, eventually. The ways to strengthen willpower constitutes one of the basic principles of improving lifestyle and therefore longevity. Most people become nervous or tense when something that is important to them needs to be achieved. Any action that is performed in this anxious atmosphere does not receive the power of the universe to support it. On the contrary, if an action is done with a calm mind and a well-made plan well and is executed with a very strong effort the universe or god supports you to achieve the desired. Without the exertion of willpower, you would simply be a machine. When Jesus said, 'Not as I will, but as thou wilt', he was also meaning the same - that we must learn to bend our will, should the will of universe or our life force be against it. Willpower, when tied down with anxiety certainly does not produce any results. On the contrary, it produces the negative feeling that we can't do it and discourages us from even attempting it because of self-doubt.'

'Can we exert the force of our will to overcome the COVID situation, guruji?' asked Stella.

'Let me ask you a question, Stella. What is will?' asked guruji.

I thought that it was a really good question. What is will?

We speak about having a strong or weak will, but what is will?

Guruji continued, 'Will is simply right and persistent prayer and action wherein we put our entire heart and mind. It is important to understand that our prayer must be legitimate. So, to overcome the COVID situation, we must cast away our mental and physical laziness and put the force of our will to overcome it.'

Stella and I agreed after this conversation with Guruji that if the Harrisons really wanted to learn more about all of this, then we should ask them to make a request in all sincerity to guruji to join in the conference call rather than audio recording it. If they were to ask us questions, we would attempt to answer them to the best extent of our learning.

We therefore decided against any recording.

5

Importance of Knowing Axis of life!

Guruji seemed to be in a jovial mood the next day on the call. After we had exchanged greetings and settled down, he asked, 'Now that you know that your present birth could be a rebirth to take certain lessons and fulfill the unfulfilled desires of earlier births, what your next question would be?'

I asked, 'Why are we born in this world? Why are we born at a particular time and place and to particular parents?'

Guruji smiled, 'The answers to these questions are not as straightforward as we'd hope.'

'Science has an answer to your first question. It says that we are born because of a combination of the alkaline sperm of a man and the acidic egg of a woman. It does not have answers to the other questions. Science does not believe in the concept of a soul taking birth and so does not even feel the need to delve into why someone is born at a particular place or time or to a particular set of parents.'

'In fact, no religion other than Hinduism answers these

questions perfectly. Hinduism says that a soul takes birth depending on its accumulated karma. The soul chooses the exact conditions, including the place and time and even the exact set of parents that will help it to exhaust the accumulated karma.'

'Hinduism also says that there are three bodies that a person has - the physical or gross body, the intellectual or mental body, called *budhi*, and the causal or atomic body, which is the reason for our birth to exhaust our deficiencies.'

'The soul takes birth on account of three debts that it owes. The first debt is that which the soul owes to the *devas* or godly persons. This reflects in the causal or atomic body. The second debt, the soul owes to its parents. This is reflected in the physical or gross body. That is the primary reason why the body has the DNA of the parents. It is "due" entirely to the parents or "owes" it entirely to its parents. The third debt, the soul owes to the rishis or scientists that it had been following in its earlier births. This is reflected in the intellectual or mental body.'

'But what is the soul? Why cannot anyone see it during birth or death? The whole misunderstanding about the soul arises because people think of it as a part of the body, which it is not.'

'Hindu scriptures say that the soul is never born and never dies on its own. So, then, what is it?'

'The soul is a part of the unlimited energy block that we spoke about earlier. It is manifested along with the three bodies that we think of as one. It does not act or react, but helps

the three bodies to indulge in actions, reactions, and doing all the worldly functions to exhaust them.'

'So, if you were to look at it from a different perspective, the soul or binding energy is here to exhaust the lessons of the causal body through the actions of the mental and physical bodies.'

'But, what are these lessons? These are nothing but the feelings of our causal body, the exhaustion of which is the main purpose of rebirth. These feelings give rise to the different chemical compositions in the body, which are essentially connected to the source of energy known as the soul.'

'What are these feelings, guruji?' asked Stella, spellbound.

Guruji sat for a while, with his eyes closed. I got a feeling that we were about to enter the realms of some profound wisdom. Guruji's eyes opened and in his calm voice, he continued, 'There are many feelings, which I will now attempt to describe. The first among them is Desire or lust. Man has unlimited desires. When one desire is fulfilled, another takes its place. The endless ocean of desires can never be fulfilled. We have to learn this lesson in life and let go of our desires.'

'The next feeling is anger. We think that whatever we say should be acceptable to others. When that does not happen, we get angry. We must learn to exhaust this feeling.'

'The next feeling is greed. Greed can be of several types, not just greed for money. This must be exhausted as well.'

'Then comes attachment. We must learn that all things are temporary in nature. So, to get attached to them excessively is foolish.'

'Pride is the next feeling. People can take pride in several things, including their riches, physical strength, beauty, or

political power. But a rich man can grow poor overnight if the stock market collapses. A physically strong man can be brought to his knees by a disease. Age diminishes beauty. History teaches us that a king could lose his crown, and sometimes even his head, in a political coup. So what do we have to be proud of? Pride is another feeling that we must learn to exhaust.'

'And finally there is jealousy. When we see someone else creating "worldly" success, we feel jealous of that person, completely forgetting that the circumstances of his life, including his "worldly" status, are simply the means to exhaust his karma. This feeling of jealousy must also be exhausted.'

'Let me tell you the story of man – let's call him Harris – who lived in the US in the 1930s, during the Great Depression. As you know, unemployment was rampant and food was scarce and Harris suffered, like many others. He beseeched God to give him money just enough to eat one meal a day. It was not like Harris had no possessions at all. His father had left him a small strip of barren land. Harris hated his father the most for this one deed that the old man had done. 'Why? Why, dad, did you leave me this wasteland?' he screamed through his tears as he prayed to God for deliverance. It so happened one day that Harris was digging about in this wasteland. For what, we shall never know. The very fact that he was even out and about in that piece of land was by itself a matter of great surprise. Perhaps it was the good deeds of a past life or even those of his forefathers that Harris struck gold that day. And I mean this literally. He actually found gold on his land. Fortune smiled upon that unfortunate man and within no time at all, he became rich. Suddenly, the same man

who had begged god for just one square meal a day was now not satisfied even with three. His wants did not stop with just that. He now wanted a good house to live in. When he had the house, he wanted the most beautiful woman in the town to be his. So the wants kept increasing. This is called lust.'

'But, guruji', I asked, 'aren't these things that every man or woman would desire?'

'There is a big difference between wanting your basic needs fulfilled and wanting just for the sake of it. In the former case, you want only enough to keep your body and soul together. In the latter case, there is no end to your wants. The interesting thing to note is that you may already have enough to live comfortably and no amount of extra possessions would be capable of making you more comfortable by even a small degree. But lust will keep you wanting more and, therefore, forever unhappy. Before I continue with Harris' story, I must elaborate my point with another small story.'

Stella and I gathered up, eagerly, to listen to this new story.

'It is said that there was a man in India, long ago, who happened to meet a yaksha in a forest. A yaksha is one of the many heavenly beings that grace the heavens of Indian mythology. Yakshas have the ability to grant you your wishes. Sure enough, that happened in this case as well. The yaksha granted the man seven jars of gold coins. The man's happiness knew no bounds. Thanking the generous yaksha profusely, he gathered his newfound, priceless possessions and ran home. We shall not debate how he gathered all seven jars in his arms and ran home with the load, because that is beside the point. We shall pick up the story after he had

reached home and eagerly started uncovering one jar after the other. True to what the yaksha had said, six of the pots were filled to the brim with gold coins. With unadulterated joy bursting out of every pore of his being, the man opened the seventh jar. As soon as he did that, his joy evaporated, for this one was only half filled with gold coins. He tore his hair in despair, cursing his misfortune and even the yaksha who had shown such carelessness in filling up this last jar. But, he was a resilient man. Wiping away his tears, he rose, determined to fill that last jar with gold. He sold a part of the estate that his father had left him. The gold coins that he got out of the transaction, he deposited into the seventh jar. To his great shock, the jar remained incomplete. From then on, filling up this unfilled jar became the aim of his life. He sold his entire possessions one after the other and deposited the gold into this jar. But, the jar remained unfilled. Within no time, in spite of the fact that he was the owner of six full jars of gold, this man was driven to madness out of despair.'

'The jars represent our wants. We may have achieved what we need, as the six full jars represent, but we always lust for something more. In the process, we end up destroying what happiness we may already have in life.'

'Now, coming back to Harris, who we had left wanting to marry the most beautiful girl in town. This damsel was called Elizabeth. Unfortunately, for Harris, Elizabeth happened to be an educated woman. This was in stark contrast to his illiterate self. This single fact was enough for her to reject his proposal. Never one to take a slight such as being rejected by the girl that he had set his eyes upon, Harris exploded in rage and pulled out the revolver that he had fallen into

a habit of carrying around to kill Elizabeth. Fortunately, he had not gone to Elizabeth's house alone. His cronies, who hung around him at all times, had accompanied him on his amorous quest. These cronies, useless at the best of times, came handy at that moment. Pouncing upon the raging Harris, they managed to knock the weapon out of his hands before he could pull the trigger. And thus a disaster of epic proportions was averted. Had Harris been able to vent out his fury, Elizabeth would have been dead and Harris himself would have had to spend a lifetime behind bars. Anger, therefore, is a feeling that needs to be exhausted.'

'You'd think that Harris would have mended his ways after that incident. But, unfortunately, that was not the case. Having struck gold on his own land, he turned his eyes toward his neighbor's land, reasoning within his greedy mind that there might be gold to be found there as well. He offered to buy them out. When they refused, he did all he could to displace them, including hiring goons to throw the people out. That was greed rearing its ugly head and making him indulge in the karma of hurting others. Greed is another feeling that needs to be exhausted.'

'Harris eventually married another woman and they had a son named Chris. Harris was devoted to this child of his. As the boy grew up, so did Harris' love for him. He was so blinded by this love that he simply could not see any fault in the boy. In all acts, fair or unfair, Harris stood by his son. Needless to say, this blind love spoiled the child, who grew up to be an arrogant young man. His head swelling with pride, Chris swiftly declined into a life of waywardness. He, however, had nothing to fear from the law, because his father's

army of lawyers was ever available to bail him out of any situation. One day, however, Chris did something that even the best of the lawyers could not bail him out of. So, did his pride last? Pride is a feeling that needs to be exhausted.'

'Chris eventually got out of prison. Being the son of a rich man, his misdeeds were even forgotten by the society. His "circle of friends" welcomed him back into their fold. In this circle was a young man named Dennis. Dennis' father was among the pioneers of the oil and gas finds in the US. As the world rapidly moved toward industrialization, oil and gas became the new hot property. Dennis' father rose rapidly to be among the richest businessmen in the country.

Dennis now had bigger mansions and better cars than anyone else in his circle of friends. This made Chris jealous of him. Soon, the feeling of jealousy took complete possession of Chris and he quarreled with Dennis. The same group of friends that had hung around his coattails now shunned him in favor of the richer Dennis. Chris slunk into the shadow of his jealousy and was soon consumed by it. Soon came a time when Chris' mind and body was ravaged by diseases. So what good did jealousy do to him? Jealousy is another feeling that must be exhausted.'

'Had Harris or Chris learnt their lessons and not done the things that they did, they would not have created any karma for their unfulfilled desires. But the chemicals and unfulfilled desires in them kept acting as impelling tendencies and eventually compelled them to act the way they did in their lives. The result was that they continued to be trapped in this cycle of birth and death.'

'The way in which these feelings manifest in you gives rise

to your karma as compared to another person and are the cause of rebirth. These feelings also create different types of diseases, as we shall see later in our discussion.'

'There is one more feeling that we must mention here. It is the feeling of fear, which destroys the self and is another cause for rebirth.'

'When a person dies with any or all of these feelings or thoughts then a rebirth has to take place in another body. This gives the soul another chance to exhaust them. Whether the soul takes a human or animal birth depends upon what it has to exhaust. However, the final exhaustion can only happen in a human birth. A soul and its unexhausted feelings survive even after a person dies. Subsequently, at an appropriate time and place when the planets can give that soul an appropriate body to exhaust those feelings, the soul is reborn in this world. Thoughts are energy. Thoughts and the soul, which is the binding energy, are not lost even when the body dies. They remain in the universe. The causal body generates these thoughts into the mental body and then the physical body acts upon them.'

'This cycle of birth and death goes on until these feelings are completely exhausted.'

'So, guruji, is there no way to end this cycle unless all the feelings are exhausted?' I asked.

'Yes, there is. Renunciation is a way to break this cycle. We shall learn about this as well when the time is right.'

'Guruji, does renunciation mean that we leave everything in this world?' asked Stella.

Guruji answered, 'the aim of renunciation is self-realization. Renunciation is often misunderstood as leaving the

world or ignoring our earthly duties. Renunciation is the process of understanding our feelings and systematically letting them go, while still continuing to live happily without fear and disease.'

'But, guruji', I asked, 'can't we exercise the power of our will to control our feelings?'

'That's a very good question, John. The willpower of a person is born out of the seat of the mind or the mental body. It can hold back or even nullify the tendencies of the physical body to some extent. So, you can see that by regular exercise and eating the right kinds of food, you can control diseases in the physical body and balance the energies also. The willpower can also to some extent control the mental body which takes the decisions that could land you into trouble. But, the will is overpowered by the causal body if it goes against the feelings with which the person was born and with which the person is attached with the energy sources. Therefore, willpower has little impact on the causal body. The unfulfilled thoughts of the causal body remain the cause of reincarnation. The only way to exhaust these unfulfilled feelings is by self-realization. That should be one of our goals in this life and one of the most potent reasons for us to live happily and longer.'

'What is self-realization, guruji?' I asked

'Self-realization, as the term implies, is to know your real self. It is to know the reasons for your birth. Once you know yourself and get out of the delusion of your present identity with this body, you would have attained self-realization. It basically means that you know that this body's identity is not real. Your real identity is the impressions or feelings in the

causal body combined with conscious energy. Once you recognize those feelings and impressions, you can let go of them. This is self-realization. In Hinduism, we follow a path of ashtang yoga or the eight habits to be able to achieve self-realization.'

'What are these eight habits, guruji?' asked Stella.

'The first habit is called yama or self restraint. It is also known as forbearance and behavior or attitude. Now we all understand possibly as to how attitude changes lives. A man with a positive attitude of love, joy, faith, and forbearance will respond differently to any situation including corona than a man with fear, anxiety of future will? The situation will prevail for some time but it is our own mind's attitude that we live happily during these times as well. Scientifically it is proven that a positive attitude increases our body's immunity, makes us popular in society, and possibly makes us more successful. The second habit is called niyama, which is our personal discipline. Self discipline is first doing things in moderation. We have seen lives getting wasted on account of addictions. It also means that there should be a set routine be it for exercising, work, pleasure, sleep, or even eating. This creates expansion of mind and visualizing abilities. The third one is aasana or seat and yoga. This is widely followed now as a health measure, but it also encourages self discipline and the quieting of the mind. The benefits of yoga in terms of a better health by increasing blood flow to all important organs of the body and not allowing fat to deposit needs no explanation The fourth habit is pranayama, which is a breathing exercise that I shall describe in greater detail a little later in our conversations. The breathing exercise helps one to really intake

oxygen in the body in a regulated manner and for maintaining flow of temperature. The fifth one is called partyahara, or withdrawal of the senses. This exercise is really the beginning of a different seeking quest. The first four habits were more to help the body but from the fifth habit begins the journey to master higher achievements. This increases the power of the mind. When we use our senses we get involved in all the worldly matters. By withdrawing we start to see the world more as an observer. The sixth one is called dharna or concentration of the mind. The purpose is to make your mind stronger. This increases your intuitive abilities and success is better achieved in the world while maintaining inner peace. The seventh one is called dhyana or meditation. Whatever I say about meditation will fall short of the advantages of meditation .It has to be experienced. It creates the magnetic power of a person and gets insights which can never be understood otherwise. The eighth habit is called Samadhi or absorption, or remaining in a state of non attachment forever. This is the ultimate experience. The entire science of the universe can be understood if one can attain Samadhi. It also gives supernatural powers to the mind.

Great importance is thus given on these eight habits and if one is able to adopt them even partially in one's life the bliss and pleasure of life felt will be of a different level.

Once we master these habits, then we become all powerful and the mind can then make anything happen in this world. However this is easier said than done, which is why it is difficult to attain godliness. The bible says, 'Thou shalt love the lord thy god with all thy heart, and with all thy soul, and with all thy strength and with all thy mind, and thy neighbor as

thy self. If you follow these precepts, then you will be able to practice the eight habits described by me to realize the self.'

Guruji paused here, knowing that we'd need time to adjust to the heaviness of the discussion that we had just had. Sure enough, he said, 'I think it may be a good idea to change this heavy discussion of meta physics, which is usually for the very hard seekers and come back to simpler ways of understanding the life forces.'

'We were talking about the significance of the planets and their influence on the human being before we branched off on this deep discussion. Do you now see the significance of the planets? The planets are the ones that decide the appropriate place, time, and circumstances for a soul to be reborn to exhaust its feelings.'

'This is the axis of life, which is unique to everyone that's born. It helps us understand the principal lesson that we need to exhaust and which will help us to end the cycle of birth and death. The most important goal in a person's life should be to know the axis of life so as to become free and to get success in this life and beyond. It is said that once we know it, accept it, and follow it, we will become more peaceful and all our efforts at renunciation will come easily to us. Therefore, the importance of the axis of life is unparalleled.'

'The other practices described in the religious texts are the knowledge of the Supreme, called gyana yoga, and the practice of love, affection, and service, known as bhakti yoga, or devotion. The combination of knowledge, devotion, and a meditative state that creates thoughtlessness or emptiness can generate an overpowering positivity. This, in turn, can help

us renounce the feelings of the causal body and make the energies more balanced.'

'Thoughtlessness!' I wondered, aloud.

'Thoughtlessness is significant, John. Thoughts create karmas and, unless exhausted, create a reactive karma which one has to undergo. You will experience the karmas of the physical body and mental body in this life. But the karmas of the causal body may have to extend to many lives unless they are exhausted or a stage of thoughtlessness is reached.'

Stella, who had been listening with rapt attention, asked, "Are the three bodies that you described inter-linked? Could you please explain them to us in greater detail?'

Guruji replied, 'your question is natural, Stella. I can understand your curiosity to know more about the three bodies and how they are different from each other. I will describe these three entities separately. However, at this stage, let us understand that it is the causal body that produces thoughts in our mind, the mental body that creates speech and which directs the physical body, and the physical body that creates actions. The synchronization of the three - thoughts, speech, and action - creates a harmony and results in a better, happier life.

In Sanskrit there is a saying, which when translated to English reads - As is the mind so is the speech; as is the speech so is the action; there is uniformity in the mind, diction and action of the noble.'

'But, people act in a manner that is exactly opposite to this precept. What they think they do not speak and what they say they do not do. This is doubtless for their selfish fulfillment, but what they forget is that this creates its own karma.'

I thought about this for a while, even as guruji took his customary pause to let the ideas to sink in. I thought of something and proceeded to question guruji, 'Guruji, we sometimes have to act contrary to this precept. Sometimes, we may know in our hearts that a person is bad, but are compelled to behave well to him. So, how can this alignment of thoughts, speech, and action be achieved?'

Guruji smiled and replied, 'I know that people think of this as the smartness that is required to survive in the world, today. But, you must understand that these karmas bring bad results in your life – diseases, quarrels in families, accidents - are all results of these karmas. So diplomacy, where you don't lie or speak half-truths, could be a possible way out.'

'Thoughtlessness can be achieved when you realize that you have no business judging anybody. That is not your job. You must realize that the person you are judging is simply acting according to his karmas of this life. There are only two categories of people – one that has the knowledge and the other that is ignorant about it.'

'Our reactions to the conduct of other people alter dramatically when we have the knowledge. When this happens, we lead a normal life full of positivity without seeing any negatives.'

Stella piped in, 'this is certainly more difficult than you make it sound, guruji. I mean, aren't we all always judging people?'

'What you say is true, Stella. But please remember that we will delude peace if we do not understand and accept this knowledge. Without inner peace, we will not know bliss and happiness. We may acquire material comforts all our lives,

but to find this inner peace, we will need to understand the knowledge that I just spoke of.'

After the customary momentary pause, guruji continued, 'I haven't forgotten about your question on the three bodies, Stella. I will answer that in detail. But, that will have to wait until tomorrow.'

Stella and I had no objection to this. As it is, we had a lot of information to reflect upon from our conversation that day.

Guruji signed off, saying, 'What is relevant is self discipline, calming the mind, and learning to look beyond our physical identity that we are known by in this world. We also need to understand how this knowledge will help us to lead a healthy and happy life and fight the COVID – 19 pandemic.'

I thought that guruji winked at me when he said that last thing about COVID, but I couldn't be entirely sure.

6

Knowing the Three Bodies and Disease Control on the Physical Plane!

Stella and I had a longer than usual conversation at lunch the next day. We spoke of the many times that we had fallen prey to the "feelings" that guruji had spoken about the previous day. Anger, greed, and pride no longer seemed like something that only happened to others. It all seemed very real. The best thing was that there seemed to be plausible explanations for why we felt each of these feelings.

'Have we ever consciously tried to exhaust any of these feelings, John?' asked Stella.

'I'm not sure about the "consciously" part, but there have been times when I have tried to get a grip on my anger. There have been times when I have tried to understand the other person's point of view.'

'But, the fact that these feelings exist, does it mean that we are carrying something forward from a previous life? I mean, have you been able to wrap your head around that whole rebirth thing?'

I had to admit that it was a difficult concept to grasp. But it did seem logical to me. Could we simply write off everything that happened as mere coincidence? What if we were actually carrying forward the burden of unfulfilled feelings from previous births? Wasn't it our duty to try and exhaust it in this birth?

Somewhere, deep inside, was also the gnawing feeling that we had perhaps run out of time or were rapidly running out of it.

The conversation that evening began on a relaxed note. It was perhaps guruji's way of easing us into the discussion after the heavy dose of learning that had been injected into us the previous evening. We talked about an evening that we had spent together on the banks of the Ganges. There were several others and it was incredible to think that guruji remembered us being there as well. The strains of the musical instruments that had been playing around us and the gentle gush of the wind as it blew over the holy river were still fresh in our minds. Our mind memorizes events that have left a lasting impression on us, guruji told us. Similarly, the other organs of the body also memorize specific feelings or impressions of the causal body. He then eased into the topic of the day.

'We spoke about the three bodies - the physical body, the mental or intelligent body, and the causal. All of them are interlinked. Let us now see how.'

'The physical body represents our health.

The feelings represent the seven organs of the body.

Desires are represented by the pancreas.

Anger is represented by the liver.

Greed is represented by the heart.

Attachment is represented by the lungs.

Pride is represented by the small intestines.

Jealousy is represented by the large intestine.

Fear is represented by the kidneys.

These seven organs are controlled by the mind. So, the mental body drives them all.

As explained earlier, the feelings drive the mental body and this, in turn, drives the physical organs. So, diseases are caused when we are not on the right path to exhausting our feelings.

Therefore, one way to cure these diseases is to get a better hold on our feelings and correct them. But, this is easier said than done.

There are many healthy habits, which, if followed regularly, also give better control of the organs and thus our feelings. They may not help us to exhaust them totally, but they would at least help us control them better.

Similarly, there are many mental habits, which, if followed correctly, help us to control, if not exhaust, the feelings and thus cure the physical body.

Needless to say, there are also many spiritual habits, which, if followed correctly, correct shortcomings that are driven by physical or mental feelings.

So, it's a two-way street. You could drive up from physical to causal via mental or down from causal to physical via men-

tal. The purpose of both journeys would be the same – to control your organs and diseases and clear the mental and causal bodies. We'll study these processes in greater detail, later, but there is no question as to the fact that spiritual practices clear all three more effectively. Good mental practices clear the physical body effectively and may also have a positive effect on causal feelings. Similarly, good physical practices may have some impact on both mental and causal bodies, but will not clear these bodies as effectively as spiritual practices. There can be no doubt that spiritual practices are superior to mental practices, which, in turn, are superior to physical practices.'

'Guruji, we would like to understand these better. But, would it be okay to start with the physical body first?' I asked.

Guruji answered, 'the cures of the physical body are also dependent upon the mental and spiritual body. So, we have to understand all of them. Nevertheless, I will first describe the path to physical cures.'

'Various sciences, such as homeopathy, ayurveda, and unani, have focused on how to improve the physical body. Let's take the example of homeopathy, first. This science was created by a German scientist, De Hennaman. Principally, homeopaths believe that all diseases flow out of the mind and thoughts. If we provide micro-atomic versions of the thing that can cause the disease itself, we will end up creating antibodies in the body, which will then help the body to fight the disease.'

'The science of ayurveda is a part of Indian herbal and metallic science. The unani system of medicine originated in Greece and probably came to India with the invading Greeks

or through the various other means of contact that the two ancient civilizations had. It continues to be practiced to this day in India too. The natural system of medicines is to eat and live as per the laws of nature to cure the disease. Specific heat or cold therapies are also practiced here. The Tibetan system works on the mind and body to improve self-expression, emotional reparation, conflict resolution, and transformation. The Chinese medicine relies on acupunctures to increase the blood flow, along with taichi practices and some herbal medicines.'

'The modern medical practices involve the use of chemical compounds to get rid of a particular situation. These medicines have the most side effects and often give rise to some other conditions. Modern medicine is the easiest to practice in today's world. That explains its immense popularity. However, the other systems have their own advantages as well.'

A disease manifests itself when there are obstructions to the blood flow to an organ. Blood circulation can be obstructed by the wrong kind of foods that we consume and which, while digesting, leave a lot of ash-like residue in the body. The thoughts on our mental plane also are responsible for the release of excess acidic enzymes in the body, other than the secretions from various glands. These also are responsible for creating extra ash which later becomes mud or mucus in the body.'

'We know that various types of acids are released in our stomach for digesting the alkaline or acidic food that we eat. After the reaction of digestion, the residue is a substance that is not soluble in water and cannot be excreted out of kidney or not slippery enough to be not able to get into our feces.

These substances get into the blood sooner or later and then get deposited in some organs, arteries, or veins in the body. Think of the chemicals released in the stomach during digestion as fire, which burns the food. The residue is ash, which is slightly thick and muddy and eventually gets deposited somewhere. Doctors have termed these deposits as fat. A naturopath calls it mucus. Practitioners of ayurveda call it kapha. Science calls it calcium carbonate or some other compound of calcium.'

Guruji paused while we digested (pardon the pun) this information. 'The body stores its minerals in the bones and the acids get released from the liver to digest food. The food could be either alkaline or acidic or a mix of both. If we consume alkaline food, the acids react with the food and produces energy. On the other hand, if we consume acidic food it simply adds to the acid already present in the stomach. This draws minerals from the bones to produce energy and depletes the mineral reserve of the body. If there is a high amount of sulfuric acid in the stomach, it will react with zinc and produce zinc sulfate and water. If there is an excess of hydrochloric acid in the stomach, then it will react with calcium, sodium, or potassium, creating deficiencies of these minerals in the body.

The blood flow is mainly obstructed by the production of calcium compounds and some carbon dioxide gas, which resides as bubbles in the pathway of blood flow.'

'Is food the cause of the deterioration of the physical body?' asked Stella.

'Food is certainly one of the causes on the physical plane. So it is important to eat more alkaline food in order to con-

trol the depletion of minerals in the body and create less of carbon dioxide and calcium compounds. If you want to know how easily carbon compounds can obstruct blood flow, just think of the calcium compound called Plaster of Paris, which we use to set broken bones. Just imagine how hard that compound becomes when set. Plaster of Paris is calcium sulfate. So what we eat is what we should regulate if we wish to lead a healthier life. But, unless we are able to control the bodies on the mental and spiritual plane, food alone cannot help the physical body. Do you now see why we must look at all the three bodies, even if we are only talking about cures for physical ailments?'

'Yes, I do', I said, 'please do describe the mental and spiritual planes which are complimentary to the physical plane to keep us disease free.'

Guruji smiled. 'Let us do that in our next call.'

Next day was as bright as the previous one was, but the fear of the pandemic was now everywhere. Rumors, many of them not entirely baseless, also fanned the flames of fear. One of the rumors that were doing the rounds was that the Chinese had been eating bats and other such beings and this culinary habit was what had caused the virus in the first place. Needless to say, we were all ears for the discourse that guruji was delivering that day, as he was going to continue on the topic of food.

"Why do we need food? It is primarily to get energy. There are seven energy producing and distributing points in the body from where hormones and chemicals are secreted to nourish all cells. These points are –

The pineal glands situated at the crown point of the brain

The pituitary gland situated between the eyebrows. This is also known as the third eye point.

The thyroid gland situated at the bottom of the throat.

The heart located at the left of the upper chest.

The solar plexus situated at the junction of the stomach and liver.

The reproductive gland situated at the base and center of the anal and sexual region and called the swadisthan chakra.

The adrenaline gland situated at the end of the lower back or near the kidney and called the mooladhar chakra.

In Hinduism, these are called chakras. These chakras resonate with different colors in nature.'

Guruji showed us a table listing the colors associated with the chakras.

Chakra	Associated Color
Pineal gland	Violet
Pituitary gland	Indigo
Thyroid gland	Blue
Heart energy	Green
Solar plexus	Yellow
Reproductive	Orange
Adrenaline	Red

'As you can see, the VIBGYOR is the base of all the energy points. When we discuss diseases and cures, we will know

how these energy points help us in curing diseases. For the present, all that we need to understand is that food of a particular color on this table will enhance the functioning of the gland in the row below it. So, though violet is the color of resonance of the pineal gland, eating violet color food will enhance the working of the pituitary gland. But please remember that we are talking only of natural colors, here.'

'Ah!; exclaimed Stella, 'that's why we need to eat greens if we are to enhance the functioning of the liver!'

'Excellent deduction!' guruji smiled.

Perhaps encouraged by guruji's praise, Stella asked, 'what if some food has a different color inside?'

Guruji replied, 'the color inside matters, but not as much as the color outside if the outside skin is also eaten. If the outside skin is not eaten, then we presume that the light spectrum has travelled from outside to inside. So if the inside is white, for instance, it means that the food has an effect on all glands."

'It is not just about the color of the food, but also about the type of food we eat', continued guruji. 'Our choice of food should change with age. When we are born, the pH of our blood is almost neutral, at about 7.5. At this age and through our childhood, we need to grow cells. So, we need more acidic food and proteins till the age of twenty.'

'After that, till the age of fifty, we need medium acidic food and proteins. After fifty, the requirement for these types of food reduces significantly. Death occurs when the pH of the blood is in the range of 4 or below, causing some organs in the body to fail. So, it is important to be mindful of what we eat as age progresses.'

'Let's take an example, here. All of us are aware that non-vegetarian foods contain more protein and are more acidic. Consuming non vegetarian food until the age of twenty helps build our muscles. From then on, the meat in our diet must be replaced with fish and eggs, until we are about fifty years of age. Beyond this, one only needs to consume egg whites or fish, if one wants to eat non vegetarian food. However, as you age, it is beneficial to practice vegetarianism and also reduce the quantity of food that you consume to ensure that the quantity of acidic foods ingested is minimal.'

'As we have discussed, fruits of different colors enhance the function of different energy points. But there is also a classification in terms of acidic and alkaline fruits. All the fruits that are bitter when not ripe and become sweet after ripening are acidic in nature. Fruits, such as apples and papaya, which do not change their taste, are classified as alkaline. Vegetables are also classifiable accordingly.'

'Milk and milk products are white and therefore have the entire VIBGYOR spectrum. But, they are also classified as acidic. There is an exception here. Clarified butter, known in India as "ghee" is alkaline. This derivative of milk can be consumed at all ages.'

I was taken aback, since this was in complete contrast to all that I had been told about clarified butter thus far. I asked, 'we are told to consume unsaturated oil and avoid butter or clarified butter, as these are sources of poly-saturated fat! Aren't these supposed to increase the fat content in the body?'

Guruji smiled. 'Ghee made from cow's milk is like nectar, or Ambrosia as the Western World might want to call it. It

increases alkalinity and also provides excellent nourishment. It is superior to the unsaturated edible oils which are acidic in nature. Ghee has a beneficial effect on digestion. Apart from this, ghee improves mobility and fluidity in joints. Since the cause of death is due to the increase in the acidity of blood, it is recommended that we consume alkaline food at all ages.'

'There is another classification of food according to its taste as far as vegetables and fruits are concerned. The different tastes are sweet, sour, salty, pungent, bitter, and astringent. To remain healthy, the food we eat should encompass all these tastes in some proportion. Excess of any one particular type creates imbalance and deficiency. So it is important to eat all types of food. This helps significantly in balancing the organs. Sweet, sour, and salty foods are all known to all of us. Examples of pungent foods include onions, garlic, and peppers. Examples of bitter food include a vegetable called bitter gourd, ginger, and neem. Pomegranate and basil are good examples of astringent food.'

'By consuming foods that are appropriate for our age, we will be able to reduce the overall ash contents or calcium compounds and the carbon dioxide bubbles in the blood stream. Consequently, we will be less prone to diseases and potentially live longer. These are the steps that we can take to remain healthy on the physical plane.'

'While we are looking at food, we should definitely also comment on spices. Remember, many traders from the west came to the shores of India in search of spices in medieval times. There are many spices, which are not consumed in the US and other western countries, which have potential health benefits depending on whether they are heat producing or

cooling in nature. Many people have taken to consuming these spices as supplements. In India, we do not bother with such practices, instead choosing to add the spices to our food directly. It has the added benefit of making food more palatable, according to our Indian tastes. But, that, admittedly, is a subjective issue. Let's now talk about spices that produce heat within the body and therefore are able to melt fat or mucus in the body. Here's a list of such spices.

Turmeric, or its extracted compound curcumin, consumed with black pepper.

Cinnamon specially consumed with honey.

Mustard seeds

Cloves — these are especially beneficial for the brain, memory and Alzheimer's Disease.

Spices that act as coolants, include -

Chia seeds

Basil

Besides, these, there are certain spices which are good for the stomach and gut and act as laxatives. These are -

Asafetida, carom seeds, and cumin seeds.

I'm sure that you'll agree with me when I say that it is important to have a properly functioning evacuation system in the body. If this is not proper and the food that we are eating is creating constipation then the regular intake of these seeds, depending on our body constitution, will help us keep the physical body better.

Guruji continued, 'Before we conclude this topic of food, let us pay attention to some little hints that nature provides us as guides to the foods to eat. The shapes of some foods resemble the shapes of organs in our body. For example, wal-

nuts resemble the human brain. Cashew nuts are shaped like the kidneys. A banana resembles the male genitals. An apple is heart-shaped. Consuming these foods has beneficial health effects on the organs that they resemble.'

'In the mental and spiritual planes, there are other means to increase the longevity of life. A human being should be able to live to the age of a hundred and twenty years. A healthy body contributes significantly to the exhaustion of karmas as the three bodies - physical, mental, and causal are interlinked.'

'The purpose of food is to maintain the temperature difference between the reproductive glands and the pineal glands at a reasonable level as we saw earlier, when we were talking about the human birth. This temperature difference is what drives the heart. When the temperature in the reproductive glands reduces substantially, the heart is no longer able to function, and death occurs. This is the most natural death. The failure of organs is not as natural a death for the simple reason that if you had managed your food better and worked on the mental and spiritual planes, then this could have been avoided.'

'In ancient times, the rishis, or scientists, would reduce their requirement of food gradually and thus live longer. We shall delve deeper into this when we discuss the spiritual plane. For now, let us understand that excessive eating shortens life. So, it is essential that we eat the kinds of food that are appropriate for our age and requirement of alkalinity.'

Guruji paused and looked away from the screen as if gazing into the distance. I had begun recognizing this as a sign

that he was going to speak of something different, briefly, and then bring down the shutters on another fruitful day

I asked, 'Guruji, is food the real cause of COVID-19?'

Guruji replied, 'It is definitely one of the causes. Food, as I described earlier, has the ability to create acidic or alkaline blood.'

He continued, 'The virus is now spreading rapidly isn't it? We are now in the grips of commotion and confusion. The question on everyone's mind is "when is this pandemic likely to end?'

I sat up in anticipation.

'If you were to rely on astrology alone then this pandemic will end in September or October of 2020. But, unless the science is understood and practiced, what will you do if this virus were to resurface some years down the line?'

Then, guruji looked at his watch and said, 'let's call it a day for now.'

7

Life and Disease Control by Spiritual Plane!

I am the kind that loves my bacon and eggs. But, when Stella placed a serving of fruit and a vegetable-laden sandwich in front of me for my breakfast the next day, I did not protest. I knew that she had been imbibing the lessons from guruji and had resolved to put them into practice. We were both closing in on our forties and the discussion on food that we had the day before had hit home hard. The very thought of ingesting stuff that got deposited in the organs and clogged the systems up was now scary.

As always, we were looking forward to the call later that evening.

'Let us first understand what we can do on the spiritual plane to control the causal body and feelings. In fact, this is the most essential plane on which we can exhaust our feelings. As explained earlier, the unfulfilled feelings in this life

cause the soul to take birth in another body while still retaining those unfulfilled feelings. Meditation and pranayama are two great practices that help us to exhaust those unfulfilled feelings.'

'We spoke about "thoughtlessness" earlier. Meditation is an exercise in which you can sit in a quiet corner and create thoughtlessness in your mind. One of the ways in which you could do this is by closing your eyes and focusing internally on the pineal gland third eye point and possibly visualizing a star and light circle there. The process looks very difficult in the beginning because there is no end to the thoughts in your mind. Even if you were to narrow it down to one thought, you'll find that it pulls in one more and then one more and before you realize it, an entire procession of thoughts is marching through your mind. It is not even like a well-organized procession, which has a beauty and meaning of its own. Many of the thoughts are irrelevant. However, if you are able to establish a practice and discipline your routine, wherein you sit over a period of time and brush aside every thought that comes to your mind by simply focusing on the star and circle, you'll see that the process becomes progressively easier.'

'You'll also notice that the number of breaths you need to keep your body running may start decreasing over a period of time, coinciding with the deepening of the thoughtlessness. Daily practice, with a conscious stretching of the duration for which you can meditate can quite your mind and remove restlessness.'

'There are several other kinds of practices of meditation. One very popular practice is known as Vipasana meditation,

which is a practice that involves internalizing your thoughts and experiencing the various sensations in the body. Yet another practice involves closing your eyes and repeatedly pronouncing the word "SOHAAAAAAM" or "HAAMSAA" and resonating with this and synchronizing it with the intake and expulsion of your breath.'

'Is "thoughtlessness" actually possible, guruji?' I asked, because I was still intrigued by the whole thing. I could actually relate to guruji's example of an unruly parade of thoughts racing in random directions through my mind most of the time.

'In the beginning, the thoughts will keep coming over and over again', replied guruji, 'you will have to consciously draw your attention back to the third eye point. With continuous efforts, you will reach a stage where you will achieve thoughtlessness. Like I said, you'll also notice a significant reduction in your breath rate. If it helps you to focus, you can visualize the god of your choice within the star. When you become fairly proficient in the practice, you'll notice a natural smile coming on to your face. This is the stage of bliss, which lasts even after you have finished your meditation.'

'To be able to meditate properly, you must realize two things. The first is that you are not this body. You are just pure energy and consciousness. You may want to see your body with your internal eye before meditation. When you see your own body like a neutral observer, you'll feel disconnected from it and the body will start feeling progressively lighter. People who have achieved very high states of meditation are sometimes able to levitate, too.'

"How can I feel different from my body? Don't I feel what my body feels?' I asked.

Guruji answered, 'Let's say that I'm actually this body. Let's also say that I was to die tomorrow. If I am really this body that I am identified with, then why would people say that "guruji's body is kept in the hall for people to pay their last respects" instead of "Guruji is in the hall so that people can pay their last respects"? Come to think of it, even this worldly name or title "guruji" is given to the energy or soul that you represent. Once the energy is gone, then your mortal remains are simply "the body". So, you are not your body. Your energy is not your body.'

'The second thing to realize during meditation is that before you reach thoughtlessness, you can observe all your organs from within. You can see the temperature, blood flow, and the energy reaching the organs. This is only to make sure that you are taking care of all the organs in your body as a sense of gratitude for their functioning. But remember that the main objective is to achieve thoughtlessness. When the breathing gets progressively slower, it reduces the elements of the causal body and the bad chemicals released from various glands. It is a very important tool. You should not get tired of practicing it regularly. In time, you will get a kind of bliss which will be more precious than anything that you can hope to achieve in this world. This is the first step of renunciation.'

'The stage of thoughtlessness reduces your requirement of melatonin, which is the sleep-inducing hormone. Restlessness, anger, and sleep insomnia all are reduced.'

Meditation is a technique by which you convert your negative emotions into a neutral or positive state. We all know that negative emotions, such as anger, create stress and causes

diseases. These emotions are the biggest killers. Therefore, it is essential to control these emotions. Meditation increases the positive emotions of love, joy, generosity, trust and these emotions nurture us.

If you regularly practice meditation, you can create a certain magnetism within you by the means of a calm mind. This is a sure shot mantra for success in life. You radiate a kind of joy that has to be felt rather than described in words. If you practice meditation regularly, you will always be in a state of meditation, whether you are moving, eating, or working. This is what is called as moving meditation.'

Guruji took his customary pause. 'I can talk endlessly on meditation. This is a practice that has to be followed regularly if you want to control all feelings of desire, anger, greed, attachment, pride, jealousy, and fear. In the present situation, there is a significant amount of fear everywhere and so meditation is an exercise that you must do every day.'

'It is said that a person has a limited number of breaths that she or he can draw in a lifetime. When we run out of this quota, death happens. Clearly, then, breath is the only connection between life and death. It is also said that the number of breaths a person takes per minute determines longevity. A man generally takes between sixteen and eighteen breaths per minute when he is relaxed. This number can go up to forty when he is exercising or angry.'

'The spiritual plane also advices how to control your breath by meditation. When you are meditating, your breath rate can go down to about seven or eight breaths per minute. In ancient times, the rishis, or scientists, would sit in mediation for years together. During this period, their breath rates

would be very little and they would live to be over a hundred and twenty years old.'

'There are a number of books on meditation and pranayama. We will dwell briefly on this subject, now, emphasizing the need to indulge in this practice to work on the spiritual plane or that causal body.'

'It will interest you to know that shallow breathing is one of the main reasons for the leaking our energy. If your breathing is shallow, then the body is unable to extract tan optimum amount of oxygen from the air. Therefore, to make up for this, the body has to breathe more often. This, as we discussed a minute ago, is what reduces the longevity of life and prevents us from reaching our full potential of years on this earth.'

'Pranayama is an exercise that you can do up to two times a day to ensure that your body parts receive enough oxygen. They may be deprived of this if you are in the habit of sitting in meditation where we are hardly breathing. If there is a deficiency of oxygen, the body parts may perform below par. To mitigate the adverse effects of oxygen deficiency, it is important to do pranayama. However, it is important to understand that, with time and practice, the body will learn to run with a decreased energy requirement without affecting the efficiency of the organs.'

'To put it simply, pranayama is a process that makes you draw in a deep breath and hold it for as long as possible so that the oxygen is absorbed in all the cells. It is commonly understood that the lungs draw in breath. But the real good breath has to be drawn in and felt by an expanded stomach.'

I marveled at how simple guruji was making it all sound.

However, I knew that these exercises were difficult to put into practice. 'Are there some practices that we can follow to make these exercises easier, guruji?' I asked.

Guruji said, 'John, every new thing looks difficult at first. This is simply because the mind is not easy to control. It runs faster than the fastest thing that you may have experienced. But, mark my words, once you learn to control your mind, you will enjoy the experience of bliss and nothing in the world would make you happier.'

'However, for your benefit, I will tell you about a few other practices to achieve this. Mind you, they may look easier than meditation, but, in reality, they take far longer and require a greater effort to achieve the same level of bliss or ecstasy.'

'The first one of these practices is called devotion to the ultimate energy or god. In India we call it bhakti yoga. It is not a physical exercise. In this practice, whatever you do in life should be done as an offering to the ultimate power. We could be doing all sorts of worldly things, but they must be dedicated in the service of the ultimate source, or god. This is also the reason why the ultimate source or god is personified in Hinduism. It is easier to visualize god as a person rather than an object or simply a source of energy if you are planning to dedicate all your actions to this entity. We recognize the godliness in Jesus Christ and that's why it becomes easier to walk with him, talk to him, or live with him every moment of your life and offer every action to him. By this practice, we imbibe the godly qualities ourselves, because we desist from indulging in actions that would not be liked by Jesus. In this way, all our feelings in the spiritual plane get exhausted.'

'In Hinduism, we have many gods and their incarnations, known as avatars. It is important to look at the message or learning we receive from them.'

'We have talked about how the world was created in our earlier discussions. The Earth was mostly water, then. So, matsya, or a fish, was the first energy and the biggest survivor on earth. So, matsya became a god in Hinduism. It delivered the message of survival in the oddest of circumstances. Therefore, to survive becomes our first duty.'

'As the earth cooled down, land masses started appearing. The energy to survive in water as well as on land became very important. This godly energy was represented by koorma, or the tortoise. The message this avatar was conveying was that we need the courage to survive anywhere. Therefore, the courage to survive is the second duty which we should learn.'

'The third godly energy came in the form of the varaha, or the boar, which created more landmass out of the water. The message of this avatar was that it is important to act to survive. Therefore, to pass through difficult circumstances we need action on the ground. These three energies dealt with our survival.'

'After this, the godly energies were available on this earth to exhaust all the elements of the causal body, one by one, so that we are liberated from the cycle of life and death.'

'Following the varaha, came the narasimha, which was half man and half lion. The purpose of this energy was to exhaust the feeling of anger. How did he exhaust the feeling of anger? It is presented in a story form that there was a demonic evil force called Hirankashyapu. I realize that the name may be a bit of a tongue-twister so let's refer to him as HK.

He developed his mental powers to such an extent that he almost attained next to immortality. He could not be defeated by any one during day or night. He could not be killed inside or outside of the house, and not by a weapon so does story go. He had a son called Prahalad. For the sake of convenience, let us name him PR. Now PR was a very noble person contrary to his father and all the efforts of HK to convert PR to the demonic way of life proved to be in vain. It would be fair to say that all was not well in the HK household. The apparent nobility and piety of his son caused a great deal of distress to HK. The all-conquering demon was disappointed with his son and did all he could to make his son see reason and walk with him on the path of terrorizing all beings on earth. But all these efforts were in vain. PR openly, but quite politely, defied his father and made HK so angry that he finally decided to kill his son PR. His main grouse with his son was that PR believed that there was a greater power than his dad HK in the universe. When he was about to kill his son the greater power of universe came in the shape of a half lion and half man and he killed HK in the twilight which is neither day or night, at the threshold of his house which was neither inside nor outside the house by attacking him with his nails which was not a weapon. But during the process the half lion and half man was so angry even though he was having godly qualities that no one knew how to cool him down. PR then hugged him and through his touch cooled him down. This shows human touch and that too deep touch like hugging or kissing can cool down the fiercest of anger of an opponent. You can use it during quarrels with your spouse also that a human touch, hug is all that takes cooling down some one.

This avatar was followed by Vamana, the midget, whose purpose was to exhaust greed. This is also presented in a story form. The story goes that there was a very rich king in ancient times who had control over the entire earth. After having conquered the earth, his ambitions made him look toward the sky. Should he now look to conquer the heavens? One would think that a man such as him would be another HK. But, far from being a demonic character, this king, called Mahabali, or the Great Sacrificer, was a charitable man who was well liked by his subjects. So, no godly energy could defeat him. But it was important to stop this man, because the laws of nature were getting defiled by his ambitions. So, the universal took the form of a midget, only two feet tall, and appeared before the king when he was holding court. There the midget, called Vamana, and appealed to the charitable nature of the king, seeking to be granted whatever he wished. The great king looked at the midget and requested him to ask whatever it was that he wanted without hesitation. After all, reasoned the king, what or how much would a midget really want? Vamana asked that he be granted as much territory as he could measure with three steps. The king burst out laughing at this request and immediately granted Vamana his wish. At this, the midget started growing in size until he attained an unimaginable size. With one step he measured the earth and with the next, he measured the heavens. Then, looking inquiringly at the king, he asked, 'Where shall I place my next step, O king?' It was then that the great Mahabali realized who it was that had come to him in the form of a midget. The king bowed down and asked the universal energy to place the third step on his head. And thus the king had to surrender

before Vamana and the entire earth got released. The moral of the story is that you need gyan or knowledge to tide over greed. And for some reason one has greed beyond proportion and attainment by foul means is desired then the universal energy brings it down. You must earn and become wealthy. But if you have too much of greed, then it can only be controlled with gyan or knowledge. One day each of us will die and we will carry none of what we unnecessary accumulate. Therefore don't live a life of greed as it may you into trouble with universal energy.'

'Then came the energy of Parashurama, the warrior, to exhaust desires. This is also presented in a story form. Essentially for cutting desires you have to shed attachment but we are not able to do so. Parashurama was a great warrior who could defeat anyone. He was very devoted to his parents. One day his father got very upset with his mother because she had some wild fantasies with someone other than him. Back in those days, women were required to be chaste even in their thoughts. No woman was to even think about another man, other than her husband. Parashurama's father was a great rishi and he could read his wife's thoughts. One should be grateful that people do not have these abilities nowadays. But, we are also much more educated and women and men are now considered equal, as they should have been always. Anyway, returning to our story, Parashurama's father was livid with his wife and ordered Parashurama to behead his mother. If he refused to carry out his father's orders, he would have to fight his father and nobody who fought Parashurama would survive. If he obeyed his father, his mother would be dead. So, it was a Hobson's choice, really. Parashurama wanted

both his parents to live, obviously. So with his gyan or knowledge he knew that he had to cut his attachment to the desire and then act. In the story, Parashurama agrees to behead his mother but, in return, asks his father for a boon. The great scientist rishi, his father, grants this to his son. Parashurama then beheads his mother. When the sage sees this, he calms down and asks Parashurama to ask what he wants in order to redeem his boon. Then Parashurama asks his father to bring his mother back to life. The Hindu stories have visualized such surgeries to have be accomplished even during those times. In that way, he manages to save both parents. But even the act of beheading his mother would have been tough for Parashurama, unless he had managed to use his gyan or knowledge to cut the attachment he felt for her. So when desires trouble your mind, you must detach from it. You can pray for it, but if there is attachment then you will be disappointed if you don't get it and then your own life will be miserable.'

'Then came the energy of Rama, the Hindu god, to exhaust pride. Rama was a very disciplined son of a peaceful king. Ravana, a powerful king of the demons, was then ruling over a vast kingdom. One day, Ravana who had heard of the beauty of Rama's wife abducted her and took her away to his kingdom. The distraught Rama put together an army of forest dwellers and took on the might of Ravana in his own kingdom. The universal energy was with Rama and he killed Ravana. The moral of the story is that you will have to fight pride or proud people. There is no other way out. The universal energy will support you.

Rama was followed by Krishna, an avatar of the universal

energy whose message was to drive away jealousy. Jealousy was brewing in the hearts of the Kauravas for their cousins the Pandavas. The Kauravas unfairly wanted to usurp the kingdom of the Pandavas and this, eventually, led to war between the two forces. Krishna was wooed by both sides. Krishna refuses to take a combative role in the war, but agrees to act as a counsel to one side that would choose him. To the other, he offers the services of his entire army. Eventually, the Kauravas chose to have Krishna's armies while the Pandavas chose to have him on their side. The story says that because of the wise counsel and intuitiveness of Krishna, the Pandavas won the war and got back their kingdom. The conclusion is simple. Wisdom and counsel is more important than the most advanced army of the world. We also learn that if you are on the right side of universal energy you will be able to eliminate jealousy.'

'Finally came the energy of the Buddha to exhaust all fear.

It is said that death is the biggest fear a human being has. We are all seeing it in present COVID world. Buddha pointed out that life and death are constantly going on, even within our own bodies. Don't cells die every minute? Aren't as many cells reborn as well? So why should one fear when all the cells in the body die when death finally occurs? Buddha proved that fear can be overcome with knowledge, meditation, and accepting the reality of life.'

Guruji said, 'All these stories are the ways to understand and increase our devotion to the universal energy, By imbibing these stories and learning from them, we are able to imbibe these qualities personified by the universal power in each story and make them our own.'

'This was not easily understood by the common people. The stories of the universal energy avatars were mainly created to present this concept in the form of stories so that even the commonest of people could access and imbibe the lessons that each one taught. Is it a wonder, then, that these avatars became gods in Hinduism?'

'Listening to these stories or reading them over and over again brings us in sync with the godly qualities that each avatar portrays. It is said that devotion to these godly energies is one way to exhaust all the elements in the causal body.'

'This is called Bhakti yoga in Hinduism. Acting according to the examples set by these godly energies will exhaust and purify the three bodies.'

'We have spoken of meditation and devotion. The third pathway is acquiring knowledge or Gyan. We all are aware that the earth is but a temporary home for all that are born here. Yet, we consider this permanent and seek ownership. Mighty kings and powerful presidents have all come and gone, staying for brief periods on this earth. Knowing the temporary nature of life and reminding oneself constantly about that fact is called Gyan, or real knowledge. The knowledge that you are not this body but energy born with a bundle of unfulfilled feelings, which you'd need to strive to exhaust then becomes the primary goal in life.'

Stella, who had been strangely quiet through most of this discourse, suddenly asked, 'guruji, John and I may have different feelings to exhaust in this life. So how shall we, as a couple, be able to exhaust them?'

Guruji smiled, 'the very reason that both of you are a couple is that there are some lessons that both of you will learn

in this life together. These lessons may have different meanings to each of you, individually, and some acts which you will do independently will draw other lessons based on conjectures of your life together. You have known that karma, as explained earlier, will impel each of you to take those lessons separately while living together. There could also be some karma that you will exhaust toward each other. In all of your worldly duties there will be some gyan, or knowledge. Knowing this worldly knowledge, which we consider as natural duty in our roles as sons, daughters, husbands, wives, fathers, mothers, brothers, sisters, or the members of the society is called dharma or religious duty in Hinduism. If we have this knowledge we don't have grief and so thoughtlessness is achieved because no reactions take place.'

'Another pathway is to do your rightful duty without any attachment and consideration as to what the outcome of your action would be. The key word here is "rightful duty". In other words, this philosophy states that if you do your rightful duty, the outcomes will take care of themselves. This is also a practice to exhaust feelings. In this practice, any action of ours is done rightfully without thinking if it will benefit us. Our actions are devoid of the feeling of revenge or any consideration to whether we have succeeded or failed. Actions are done just because they are right, without emotional constraints or any considerations to the outcomes of our actions. So it exhausts the anxieties of uncertainties about the future and our desires and feelings in the causal body.'

'This particular pathway or practice is what the holy book of the Hindus, the Bhagavad Geeta, is all about. It contains the very essence of Hinduism.'

'However, the higher spiritual plane is achieved when irrespective of whether your circumstances are good, bad, or ugly, you don't react and consider everything as the will of god or simply our lessons in the life. That is the height of devotion in these practices. This is called surrender to the universal energy while you continue to perform your duty. There is a great emphasis on surrender and letting go. This is a form of relaxation and emptying of the mind. When you are relaxed the muscles are open, the breathing is soft, and you connect to the higher forces of the universe.'

I will tell you a short story. This happened in East Africa, when it was ruled by the British. One day, the governor and his army commandant were sitting in the courtyard, admiring a pair of ferocious Rhodesian Ridgeback dogs that the commandant had presented the governor. Suddenly, one of the dogs broke loose and flew at the governor. Before he could react, the dog had bitten off a part of his little finger. The governor was immediately rushed to the hospital where the doctors decided to amputate his entire finger so that sepsis did not set in. When he was recuperating in the hospital, the commandant paid him a visit. The governor asked the commandant why the dog had attacked him and spared the commandant. Being a god-fearing man, the commandant answered that it was god's will and even if god causes injury to someone it is for the benefit of the victim. The commandant was in a state of surrender but the governor was not. The latter lost his temper and accused the commandant of trying to intentionally harm him. The governor ordered the commandant be arrested and imprisoned, until a proper enquiry could be made into the entire incident.

Some days later, the governor decided to go hunting, possibly to snap out of the foul mood that he had sunk into following the loss of his finger. In the deepest part of the bush, he became separated from the rest of the hunting party and was captured by a tribe of cannibals. The cannibals wanted to sacrifice him to their god. The shaman was about to chop off the governor's head when he noticed the amputated little finger. Immediately, he called a halt to the rituals. It would never do to sacrifice an imperfect man to their god. Eventually, the tribe released the governor. He was then reunited with his party, which was frantically searching for him, and made his way to safety of the cantonment.

The governor who returned to the cantonment was a changed man. He asked for the commandant to be produced before him. He narrated the incident to the commandant and said 'had it not been for the amputated finger, I would not have had the good fortune of releasing you from prison and admitting that I now see the wisdom of your words. But I have a question for you. Why did god let you suffer in prison even though you were there for no fault of yours?' The commandant smiled and replied, 'Sir, the will of god is as clear as the sky is on a summer morning. Had I not been in prison, I would have accompanied you on the hunt and as is my bounden duty, never have let you out of my sight. Needless to say, I would have been captured by the cannibals, much as you were. And finding me whole, the savages would have sacrificed me to their god. By causing me to suffer briefly, god was ensuring that I stayed alive, too.'

Guruji said, 'The power to accept that all that happens to

you is god's will and is good for you is the power of surrender.'

'The whole purpose is to control reactions, judgments, and living as ultimate energy or consciousness. Simply put, this means living in the world, but not getting attached. It means living without accumulating any karma even though indulging in duty bound actions at all times.'

'When we concentrate on the point between the two eyebrows in meditation our willpower is in tune with the universal power and the life force can bring about any changes in the body to free it from diseases, tensions, or restlessness. Therefore, it is a cure as well as a preventive tool for not getting any disease in the first place. Meditation, coupled with right living and food habits as basic laws of health, improves the super conscious state of the mind improving the intuitive state or the so called sixth sense state. This will help you get material prosperity as well.'

'There are two positive actions in spiritual science that can help us to exhaust all the elements of desire, anger, greed, attachment, pride, jealousy, and fear. These two actions can be described by the simple phrase "love all serve all". You obviously don't need this to be explained. Selfless service to all creatures of this world and selfless service to whatever they may be requiring can really exhaust the feelings. As a bonus, the satisfaction that you will derive by your actions will make you live happily. These two actions of selfless love and service can wipe off all the elements in the causal body, thus liberating you from cycle of death and life.'

Stella asked, 'But what about the times when I cannot be

of any service to my fellow human beings? There are so many times when I fall short of their expectations.'

'The thought is significant as well, Stella. It signifies that you wanted to help to the best of your ability, but fell short. This does not signify that a service was not rendered. You can make up for the shortfall in your efforts by praying to the ultimate energy to help out the person who was in need of your service. That completes the service.'

'How do you define love?' I asked.

'Respect, compassion, and the willingness to sacrifice the self for the benefit of the loved one, without any desire for being compensated for that act, is called love.'

"Today, it is very easy for many of us to say "I love you", isn't it?' asked Guruji. 'We consider attraction also as love and any relationship we define by saying I love you. The words become meaningless because we don't act in a loving manner whenever the situation is against us in our relationship. We sometimes don't help our parents since we are busy in our own pursuit of desires in life. But this is all against the universal law and therefore we don't get liberated from our feelings or impressions of the causal body. In selfless love, there is no feeling of love for the body but only for whatever the energies the other person has howsoever insignificant the person may be in our pursuit of our life.'

'The Hindu holy book of Srimad Bhagwatam depicts the characters of two godly energies, Krishna and Rama, the highest forms of energies on earth. Their life lessons can teach us how to express selfless love, how to follow discipline with love, and how to perform our rightful duties. If we follow these two godly energies, that is the science of liberation,

in my opinion. But, without doubt, there would be similar examples within the Bible and the texts and stories of other religions as well.'

I asked, 'Guruji, how do we know what rightful duty is? What is right for me may be the exact opposite for someone else.'

'That's a very relevant question', replied guruji, 'Let me tell you a story that may shed some light upon this topic. In the days gone by, there was a man named Daya, which means compassion in Sanskrit. He was often to be found meditating outside his hut in the forest. One day, while he was meditating, a merchant approached him, looking scared to death. 'Oh holy one', the merchant sobbed, 'I am being pursued by some goons hired by a rival merchant. With your permission, could I please climb this tree and hide myself?' Daya did not answer, but continued meditating. The merchant took his silence for consent and clambered up the tree and hid himself in the dense foliage. The goons that the merchant had referred to arrived shortly thereafter. In a rough voice, the goon who looked like the leader of the gang demanded, 'hey, you? Have you seen a merchant come this way?' A dilemma broke out in Daya's mind. Wasn't it his duty to speak the truth? This was immediately followed by another thought. What if he remained silent? Surely, he couldn't be accused of not speaking the truth, then. Having satisfied himself that this was the appropriate thing to do, Daya remained silent. But the goons were not to be so easily put off. They started trashing Daya with the clubs that they were carrying for purposes such as making silent mendicants speak. So zealously did they go about this task that they broke poor Daya's hand.

The one that would not speak a few moments ago was now squealing piteously on the ground. Realizing that the goons wouldn't stop until they had extracted the truth from him and that his very life was in peril, Daya decided to speak the truth. With his one good arm, he pointed to the top of the tree. Immediately, one of the goons clambered up the tree and threw the terrified merchant down. The others pounced upon the hapless man and pounded him to death. Not being satisfied with their one cruel deed for the day, they returned to their unfinished task and dispatched Daya also to the next world.

Arriving simultaneously at the gates of heaven, the two recently departed souls were ushered into the presence of a judge. Each presented his case. Daya also added how he was confident that he was on the side of truth.

To which the merchant raised an objection. He argued that he had asked Daya for permission before hiding in the tree. If Daya had no intention of protecting him, then he could have at least indicated to the merchant to go find some other place to hide. But he chose not to speak. So how could he now insist that he had done his rightful duty?

The question now was "what was Daya's rightful duty?"'

Guruji turned to me and asked, 'John, if you were the judge, what would you have said?'

I thought about it intensely. Daya had tried to keep himself out of the matter for as long as he could. Finally, what he had said was the truth. So, hadn't he done his rightful duty? But, had he acted with compassion?

Seeing the look of confusion on my face, guruji smiled, 'Your first duty is to save yourself. So, Daya failed in his duty when his actions caused him to have his hand broken.

Secondly, what good is a truth that cannot save a life? Does it serve any purpose? Could Daya not have simply pointed to a wrong direction just to save the merchant's life? Would that not have been his rightful duty?'

'The rightful duty is therefore to help. A small lie would have possibly generated an adverse karma. But compared to the karma that Daya generated by his actions, it would have been insignificant. Daya's actions cannot be considered his rightful duty.'

'So every act that you perform must be done in the light of the knowledge of your rightful duty. The rightful duty is simply the appropriate thing to do under the given circumstances.'

'Is any religion superior to the others?' I asked.

'Religions are all the same, even though they may be expressed in different forms. They all hope to achieve the same objectives.'

'The Buddha says that we are dying every moment because some of our body cells are dying even as we are sitting here speaking to each other. So, doesn't some part of our body die every second? Therefore there is nothing to grieve in this life. So take out any fear from your mind and learn this eternal truth.'

For a moment, my mind drifted to the pandemic that had begun spreading its ugly tentacles in New York. Fear was the buzzword all around. I wondered if this advice to not grieve and to banish all fear from our minds was actually something that everyone could put into practice.

Guruji continued, 'Our minds are the culprits. Unless we are able to control it and make it subservient to our present,

it will keep dreaming and planning about the future. We are not living in the present, but in an assumed world of the future as planned or visualized by our mind. Therefore, all of us must practice the spiritual plan that we discussed thus far.'

On that note, guruji closed the discussion for the day, leaving Stella and myself to ponder over all that we had learned that day.

The definition of love that guruji had given us that day continued to baffle us for a long time after the call. We talked about it late into the night. Our understanding of love thus far had been that it was a tender emotion. But the discourse had added a new dimension to our understanding. Love was where respect, compassion, and sacrifice of oneself were greater than any ideas of me and mine. If every couple was to follow these simple ideas, there would never be any conflict between them and life would be so peaceful.

And how well had guruji explained the concept of service! Stella was so taken in by the knowledge that even if she was unable to help someone completely, she could still make up for it with her prayers. Was prayer powerful enough to uplift or help the millions of poor around the world that remained untouched by our service due to our limitations? Perhaps focused prayer really did have that kind of power.

And then there was the discussion on controlling our negative emotions and releasing them. I felt a wave of excitement pass through my being when I thought of how creative I could be were I to not carry any negatives within me.

A feeling of peace was surely beginning to dawn upon me and it was a feeling as happy as I had ever experienced in my life.

8

Life and Disease Control by Mental Plane!

'If we are able to regulate our mind, then we will be able to control the physical, mental, and causal bodies.'

'In homeopathy, it is said that most of the diseases in the physical body starts from the mind alone. Therefore, homeopaths tend to treat the mind by giving very subtle atomic particles of medicine so as to produce antibodies.

'As we have seen earlier, the physical, mental, and causal bodies are interconnected and if we are able to control one we would be able to influence the others for the exhaustion of the reasons for our rebirth.'

'The mind has two important segments, the seat of intellect and the seat of ego. Most people do not understand ego and remain in denial about their own egos while acknowledging that of others. Some people cannot differentiate between self confidence and ego and argue that they have the

former and not the latter. The word "I" is ego. When you say "I can do it", that is a statement of ego as well as self confidence. But, when you say "I alone can do it" then that is ego. If there is even a hint of pride in your statement, then that is also ego.'

'Is ego bad, guruji?' asked Stella, with a meaningful glance at me.

'You need some ego to live in this world. Otherwise, there is a danger of slipping into a vegetative state. But, the ego should be so small that you should be aware of it. If you are able to control ego, then you win the war on the mental plane. Ego can be controlled through intelligence and intellect.'

'If you are able to analyze why a thought has come to your mind, you'll be able to know whether it has occurred to you because of your ego or because of some other reasons, such as attachment .If we can really develop the practice of analyzing each and every thought that comes to our mind, then we can identify the source of the feeling which is behind that thought. One of the most powerful practices in the mental plane is the continuous examination of our thoughts to negate the ego.'

'As soon as you realize the reason why a thought has occurred to you and are able to negate the feeling of "I" in that thought, then you would have controlled your ego. This is a practice that we should indulge in routinely because it will help us to stay humble, speak softly, and thus live more happily. Gratitude will automatically take roots within us if we control our ego. We shall have a nature that is liked by others and that is the power of the intellect. At any

one moment, our minds are filled almost to capacity with thoughts, feelings, memories, hopes, fantasies, fears, anxieties, projections and more. Our minds are incredibly rich with knowledge, data and experiences, lessons we've learned, conclusions we've drawn, attitudes, and reactions. So what you need to develop is controlling the "I" in all of these fillers and fill them with love, affection, courage, forbearance, and gratitude.'

'By examining every thought that comes to our mind, we will develop an ability to analyze ourselves.

At present, we are simply machines that are going through our daily routines of breakfast, lunch, dinner, work, and sleep and occasionally finding random means of keeping ourselves entertained. We don't know our life goals or what lasting satisfaction and complete happiness means. We are simply spending our lives as robots. Let us do an exercise for the next couple of days. Let us write down our thoughts and aspirations for and analyze what we are, and not what we imagine we are. Let us also think about what we want to become.

'Of course, the traits from past lives may influence us now. Also, unlike in the animal kingdom where a good pedigree animal is most likely to beget a good offspring, there is no guarantee that we will be great simply because our parents are. But, with self analysis we can change the course of life. We also must know that physical and mental aspects are interrelated. So by improving thoughts and making them positive our physical health can improve as well.'

'We must also realize that the world is what our mind makes it to be. Whether we look at a challenge as a difficulty or an opportunity to progress depends on our mind. If the

mind gets disturbed because of the acts of others or because of environmental reasons it creates negative thoughts and actions happen accordingly. So let us live with peace irrespective of the surroundings.'

'There is another quality that we have to develop on the mental plane. That quality is called faith. All religions in this world were created to develop our faith so that we don't go into depression. All religions give us the guidance to increase our faith in the ultimate power. Difficulties are inevitable in every life. Faith gives you the power to overcome and live through these difficulties.

'Have you heard of the phrase "blind faith"? Unfortunately or, perhaps, fortunately, faith cannot be blind. Faith is often misunderstood as blind. That is not a quality of faith at all. There have been and perhaps still are some cults which blindly follow the rules that the cult leaders ask them to. They do not bother to understand it using the prism of knowledge and wisdom. Let me tell you a story. In Indonesia, some years ago, lived a god fearing person named Michael. As you may remember, in 2004, Indonesia was struck by a huge Tsunami. Michael lived close to the coast and his town was one of the many that was affected by this disastrous event. Even as the town started flooding up, Michael rushed to the top floor of the building that he resided in to save himself. Being the god fearing person that he was, Michael did his rightful duty and kept praying to god to save him. Soon enough he heard the powerful motor of a navy boat coming his way. People were gratefully clambering up the boat and the vessel was filling up fast. Michael thought to himself, 'what if this boat was to sink? Look how overcrowded it already is!' Thinking so, he

sank to his knees and continued to pray to god rather than take the opportunity to save himself. Soon enough, he saw a helicopter coming his way. Someone in the helicopter must have spotted him, because a rope was thrown down. Seeing the rope swing dangerously in the air, Michael's heart pounded in his chest. He thought, 'what if I was to lose my grip and fall? Surely, I'd die. This is not my deliverance. I have always prayed to god and am doing so now as well. I have full faith that he will come to my rescue.' Thinking so, he continued to pray, thus foregoing another opportunity to save himself. Just minutes after helicopter had gone away, the building that Michael was on collapsed, taking Michael with it to a watery grave.'

'What must have happened thereafter, I cannot say. But, I'd like to imaging that he went to heaven. On judgment day, a rather indignant Michael must have confronted his creator and asked in a vexed tone, 'Lord, why did you not come to repay the faith that I had invested in you and save me?'

'To which god, in his heavenly voice must have replied, 'Twice, my son, did I send my angels your way that day. But you disregarded them in your blind faith. When you chose not to use the wisdom and knowledge that I had bestowed upon you, why blame me?'

'Faith has to accompanied by wisdom. You must be wise enough to see through the rules of cults if real wisdom prohibits you.'

'This is not to say that faith is not an important virtue. It gives you the power to move forward.'

'In Hinduism, we develop faith by discipline, fasting, and sacrifice. Discipline means a fixed pattern in all things we do

in life, right from waking up to sleeping. Fasting and sacrifice improve our will power, which is an important constituent of the mental plane, and is different from ego. Will power plays an important part in achieving our objectives in this life and beyond, and is really responsible for making our character.'

'Guruji, what should the duration of a fast be? What does sacrifice mean? I asked.

'Fasting should be done to increase the will power and for the time and frequency that your body is comfortable with. There cannot be an external imposition. Sacrifice, on the other hand, is becoming other-centered, rather than self-centered, and discarding the thoughts of me and me alone in all walks of life.'

'These are all parts of self realization. Self realization means to know your real nature. This, above all, plays an important part in knowing what you really are and not what you are known in this world as. To give you an example, the president of a country might feel very powerful because he controls the people of an entire country. But what is he in the real universe? His country may be significant in this world, but the world itself is a tiny spec in our solar system, which, in turn, is a tiny spec in the universe. The president who feels that he is "someone important" does not realize that he is only an infinitesimally tiny dot in the universe. This self realization is very important to control the ego and develop other qualities.'

'Another science that I follow to control the mental plane is astrology. I can see that you are raising your eyebrows, John, when I call astrology a science. Many people think that

it is no science and is a part of religion. I will explain why that is not the case.'

'We are all aware that a high tide is caused in the ocean when the moon comes nearer to the earth while rotating in its orbit and a low tide happens when the moon is farthest in its optical orbit of the earth. Now, if the moon can influence water in the ocean, can it not influence the water within our body? Doubtlessly, the moon influences our cells and blood, where the water within the body resides. Its relative position to the place where we are born has good or bad effects in our daily lives. The cells combined create an aura which can be photographed these days by Kirlian technology. And this aura interacts with the aura of other people resulting in a good or bad relationship or good or bad chemistry and bonding between the individuals. The cells also influence thinking and thoughts. Thus, there is a bond between the moon and thoughts.'

'Similarly, all the other planets in the zodiac, which are able to influence things on the earth, are able to influence different chemicals in the body. For example, the planet Saturn has got an abundance of iron and zinc in its atmosphere and its proximity to the earth decides how the iron and zinc chemicals in our body react. That is how Saturn influences the cells in our body and affects the aura. The aura is thus the combined resultant effect of all the planets affecting the various elements in the body and consequently the cells. The aura is the cause of all that happens to our mental plane, including money income, relationships, properties, diseases, and so on. The aura is also responsible for our luck, fame, and even the time of death.'

'You may have, by now, understood that there is a science behind the study of planets in your astrological chart and your persona. However, it is an impelling science which means that the cells put you or drive you in that direction. But if your will power is strong then you can avoid being impelled in that direction. This is the importance of will power. Please do not equate it to stubbornness or overconfidence, as will power is not easy to get. It can only be achieved with a lot of discipline, fasting, and sacrifices.

'Another reason to call astrology a science is that it is associated with behaviors. All behavioral sciences are considered as science, as a psychiatrist will tell you. Given identical circumstances, two persons may behave differently and thus there are exceptions, but, by and large, the behavior expected is well defined.'

It is also true that there are very few astrologers who practice astrology as a science. So, many scientifically-minded people have a disconnect with astrology. But those that know it as a science and the curative portion of the treatment of the defects play important roles. I give greater importance to the curative portion of this a science rather than forecasting the impelling future itself though both go hand in hand. To tell a patient that you are suffering from malaria is not good enough. The doctor must know what medicines to give to cure malaria and therefore the curative science is more important than the science of diagnosis. Therefore, in my opinion, will power works better when combined with the curative portion of the science or methods prescribed by an astrologer. Again, in my opinion, a complete change or cure is difficult to achieve because the purpose of this life, as we

have discussed so far, is to exhaust elements. Therefore, the axis of life has to be also understood. If we try to oppose it, it creates a struggle between the past and the present. It is also been my observation that there are very few astrologers who understand and can read the axis of life of a person, which is connected with why he is born in this world.'

'What is this axis of life Guruji? Could you please explain astrology so that we can understand it as a science?' asked Stella.

Guruji sighed. But we could see that he was happy with our eagerness. He said, 'That subject is very deep. It will have to wait until tomorrow.'

'In short, however the axis of life can be defined as the purpose why we are born in this life. Everyone has to exhaust some karma or feelings in this life and if those be considered as a lesson then the axis of life defines the primary karmas among all our accumulated karmas we need to exhaust and learn lessons from. To know that is a great achievement since we otherwise waste our energies in directionless, meaningless pursuits and remain unhappy.'

9

Axis of Life and Astrology!

Guruji was more cheerful than usual the next day.

'You have seen how planets influence the human aura and therefore all its actions. The planets which influence the aura are the sun, moon, mars, mercury, Jupiter, Venus, Saturn, and newly found Pluto, Uranus, and Neptune.'

'Besides these, there are two nodes that form the axis of life and in Hindu astrology are known as rahu and ketu. Western astrologers don't give much regard to these, as they have no energy or matter of their own. In Hindu astrology, planets like Pluto, Neptune, and Uranus are not taken into consideration for individuals as much, since they are very far off from the earth. They are, however, accounted for when an astrologer studies natural disasters or epidemics.'

Stella asked, 'Guruji are astrology forecasts 100% accurate?'

Guruji said, 'No, I don't think so. I had explained earlier that it is an impelling science and not compelling so it can

never be 100% accurate. However, you know your traits really and that helps you to create guides and precautions in your mind.

Guruji took a pause and asked, 'Is medical science 100% accurate?' If it was then there would be no death. There are definitely many success stories of medical science, but failures are a part of it, too. Similarly I will say there are number of success stories in astrology and there are a few instances of failure too. So it is a guide. There are astrological reasons for this pandemic also and I mentioned to you in August, last year that something was about to happen to the world in March of 2020. But did I imagine that a pandemic would hit us? Not really. And that the impact would be so severe was also beyond my abilities to comprehend. But I did see some impelling tendencies and that is what strengthens my belief in astrology.'

Guruji said that instead of focusing on the world let us first talk of individual humans

'Let us focus on individuals alone and thus disregard the distant planets. The entire life of an individual is projected in 360 degrees and divided into 12 representations of 30 degrees each. Each of these sectors are called houses. These are represented from the serial time when you are born as:-

Personality, Status, and Character — There are certain chemicals within our body that make our personality the way it is. We can change our personality, self-confidence, and status to some extent, but please do remember that some of our personality traits are the way they are to help us complete the lessons that we took our birth for.

Wealth, family, and friends - After our personality and

health, we care most for our wealth and family. We all want better bank balances and would constantly love to improve on it.

Courage, Co-born (brothers or sisters) — We need courage to achieve our wants. We also need good relations with our co-born.

Property, mother, general material home, and comfort of servants etc. - This is called the pleasures of life, since we all want good relations with our mother, good properties to live in, and good followers to follow us.

Education, intelligence, romance, intuition, and children - All of us desire high education and intelligence and, in many cases, we crave for children too.

Diseases, enemies — No one wants them but we cannot avoid them. We want to get rid of them as fast as possible. But we all see these negatives in life

Spouse, partnerships — A harmonious co-existence with your spouse is generally a feeling of happiness in this world. We even desire good relationships with our ex-spouses.

Death and life longevity, debts — No one wants death or live in debt. But we still have to pass through this to get better longevity and peaceful death.

Luck, religious nature — It is said that if you are lucky, it is good enough to get things easily in life without much effort. So everyone wants to see if they are lucky or how to increase luck.

Father, fame, occupation - people crave for fame in this world and recognition becomes a big want

Income, winning chances — without sufficient income,

even wealth does not look very good to us. So this is a must to derive satisfaction.

Expenses, imprisonment, hospitalization, and exhaustion of the elements of the causal body — this is also not liked by anyone, even though it is useful in exhausting the cycle of birth and death.

'These twelve aspects of human life are defined by the seven planets and two nodes occupying some degrees in this entire three hundred and sixty degree universe at the time of your birth. Each 3 degrees and 20 minutes define a constellation in Hindu astrology and the placement of all these nine planets in each constellation and then their subdivisions give strength, knowledge, and benefic or malefic aspects on the individual as per astrology.'

'The axis of life is defined as the constellations and degrees the nodes are positioned in at the time of birth. This is regarded as the definition as to why we are born, what our past life could have been, what the way forward to exhaust the elements for which we are born in this life should be, and how we could gain the most out of this life for which we were destined.'

'People get lost as they are often misdirected in their quest to understand this axis of life. Therefore they remain out-of-sync with their purpose in life. It is not easy to understand and accept this axis. But, we all need to do this in order to avoid unnecessary depletion and deflection of energy. To understand it, I recommend that you deal with an astrologer who understands this science very well. Like I said, most astrologers have no knowledge of this concept of life which should have been the main focus. What you need is the time,

date, and place of your birth to be able to understand all these energies flowing in your body. I have seen many people get depressed because they are unable to know their purpose of life. Without knowing the axis of life, they remain ignorant and get defeated and depressed.'

'Guruji, I have a very interesting anecdote to narrate from my last trip to India', I said.

'Go on', encouraged guruji.

'Well, it was a very novel and a bit of a hair-raising episode for all of us. Stella, Ruth, and I were at dinner at one of our acquaintance's home one evening. There were several guests, prominent among who was a hypnotist. After dinner, when we were all relaxing, our host casually asked the hypnotist if he could demonstrate his powers of past life regression. The hypnotist readily obliged and asked around for volunteers. Many guests, including the three of us, declined. But, needless to say, our curiosity was aroused. Finally, one of the guests volunteered. The hypnotist asked this man to recline on a deck chair and then put him into a semi-coma state. When he was apparently convinced that the volunteer had traveled back in time to his previous birth, the hypnotist asked him who he had been back then. To our shock, the semi-conscious man replied that he had been a priest of a Ganesha temple. Ganesha, I learned later, was a Hindu god. He went on to describe the temple in great detail, including that it was on the banks of a river that he had been fond of bathing in. Then, the story took a dark turn. Apparently, the man had been fond of gambling and had incurred a huge amount of debt as a result. Finally, in desperation, he had stolen the jewelry that adorned the deity. The theft was dis-

covered the next day and the matter was presented to the village chief. The chief guessed, rightly, that only the priest could have done the deed. But, he had a bit of a soft corner for the priest and declared him not guilty, and thus saved him from the wrath of the villagers.'

'I think that the hypnotist had had enough of the story and so he woke the volunteer up. We were astonished and also a bit uncomfortable after the session was done.'

Guruji, who had been listening calmly to my tale, smiled and asked, 'I'm sure that you have a question for me, John. Go ahead and ask me.'

'Guruji, after all that we have discussed about karma, I want to know what karma had the priest created for his next birth? What became his axis of life to learn the lessons?'

Guruji replied, 'In my view the priest would have been born as a very noble person in his next birth. This may not be surprising to you since you have already met the former priest in his present life. He would be a very knowledgeable person, but always short of money. It is also likely that his gambling habit from his previous life would be tormenting him in this one as well. He is possibly also having quite some trouble from the government of the country, regarding non-payment of taxes or such. His axis of life will be his desire to earn more and more. That cannot be achieved until he quits gambling.'

I was dumbstruck. I had become acquainted with the gentleman after his hypnotism session had been done. I had got to know that he was well educated and from a good family. But he was forever short of money and often had reached out to many of the other guests that had been present that day for

loans. He, apparently, had also defaulted on loans and was in some trouble with the taxmen.

'And what about the chief, guruji? Would he suffer any karma for his actions?' I asked, unable to keep the wonder out of my voice or eyes.

Guruji laughed. 'I think I hit the nail on the head, John. The wonder in your eyes is a dead giveaway. Well, for all you know, the chief from the past birth may have been present in that very get together where the hypnotism session took place. In his present birth, the chief may have been subservient to priest for some time because of his attachment. In all likelihood, he may have broken away by now, but will always want to help the priest even in this new birth. This is my analysis of karma and axis of life for the chief.'

'Guruji, whatever you said about the former priest's karma and axis of life in this birth is true. I have no reason to believe that that may not be the case for the former village chief, either.'

Guruji smiled, 'Well, I can only point to the general direction that his karma and axis of life might have taken in this life. But, depending upon his will power in this life, he could have added or subtracted from this result somewhere. So, a deviation might also have been possible.'

Guruji continued, returning to the topic of the curative portion of the energies. 'The curative portion of these energies, as explained earlier, will be the main focus of an astrologer so as to guide you to be able to get a better control on your mental plane. As explained earlier, we have only three energies in this universe - sound energy, light energy, and fire energy. When we use these original energies to correct

the energies that we are born with, cure happens. Combining this with will power, we believe, can cure nearly fifty percent of the malefic impact of an energy prevalent in your body. We don't find a hundred percent cure because neither do we have such strong will powers nor can we completely change the destiny of our lives, since the purpose is to exhaust certain elements of our causal body. But even fifty percent is no mean achievement! These cures do not diminish your wants, but help you to achieve them while simultaneously, over a period of time, making you realize that the principal method is to realize self and have the knowledge which creates this life. Thus the wants also diminish over time. The wants mentioned here include all the elements of the causal body be it desire, anger, greed, attachment, pride, jealousy, or fear. Individually, these could be malefic to you, but you may still want them in this life, because, without them being available, you would be unable to exhaust them.'

The customary pause was longer this time. Guruji knew that he had given us a lot to think about.

'So let me start with sound cure. This involves the chanting of individual hymns in a particular way to create sound. Multiple repetitions of these hymns cure the gland or chakra. This in turn regulates the hormones and chemical distribution in the line of wants.'

'Fire energy can be used for curing by lighting fire in a particular manner and burning the barks of some trees and other materials to create a thermal energy vapor. This cures the glands by regulating the hormones and chemicals in the direction of want.'

'Light energy cures involve making the individual wear

some specific stones on their fingers to create an electromagnetic current in particular glands to be able to regulate hormones.'

'As you are well aware, this body is run on an electromagnetic field caused by the temperature difference between the reproductive glands and the pineal glands. When you wear a stone, you are adding Eddy currents to the electromagnetic field, thus altering the electromagnetic field of particular gland, by means of which you improve your chances of getting what you want. Some of the stones used are diamonds for Venus, rubies for the sun, pearls for the moon, red coral for mars, emerald for mercury, yellow sapphire or topaz for Jupiter, blue sapphire for Saturn, cat's eye for ketu node, and garnet for rahu node.'

'It is important that you engage an expert astrologer to help you choose these stones. Most of these stones have side effects that are not understood normally. Remember that there are no free lunches! When you add some energy to change the electromagnetic field to influence a particular gland, you are also suppressing some other energy. So, this needs to be handled with utmost care.'

'In today's world, the energy cures with sound and fire are possibly clumsy and time consuming. So wearing a stone on some finger to create an Eddy current in a particular gland is perhaps the only practical answer. The fingers of our hands are connected to some energy distribution points of glands or chakras. This has been acknowledged in acupressure and acupuncture. So, the fingers and are scientifically proven to be able to carry those currents or vibrations. The purpose is

to influence the release of hormones and chemicals from a particular gland to be able to achieve a want,'

Guruji ended with a word of caution. 'To fulfill wants is the desire of all human beings. But, unless we know how to break this cycle of life and death, it will give us only material pleasure but not bliss and eternal happiness.'

Stella asked, 'Guruji, isn't material pleasure an important objective of this body? So why you are cautioning about it?'

Guruji replied, "all material pleasures one day will cease to be. When you achieve them, you derive some pleasure at first, but, after a while, the pleasure diminishes. I am, therefore, emphasizing on lasting happiness. I understand that sometimes it is essential to get the material pleasure as much in order to exhaust your wants and clear lessons of life. But it is important to remember always that these are temporary. For your benefit, I will continue my guidance to you on these material pleasures also. But, I would want to remind you that when we are in between these pleasure trips that life gets us into unwanted troubles, such as this pandemic, which cuts some of the pleasures.'

'But, that's for tomorrow. We'll see some concrete steps that you need to take to increase material pleasures using stones. We'll also see how we can cut some of the associated troubles and keep them to the bare minimum.'

10

Curative Astrology!

'As we saw yesterday, stones have a huge impact in a person's life, when that person has a want or need to achieve something. These could be prolonging of life, freedom from disease, increasing material comfort, increasing wealth, improving relationships, and even winning over legal matters and enemies. These stones are naturally-occurring precious stones. Some semi-precious stones also give results similar to some precious stones, because of a similar chemical composition. Take a look at this table. It lists the function of the stones and their chemical makeup.'

Guruji shared his screen to show us the table.

1. Ruby — Blood Red in color. It increases will power, political power, and ego. It is primarily made of chromium ions replacing aluminum oxide base. It generally denotes the sun and the soul.
2. Pearl — White in color. It increases calmness, regulates blood pressure and anxieties. It is a compound

of calcium, particularly calcium carbonate. It generally denotes the moon and the mind.

3. Red Coral — Red in color. It increases courage, physical strength, anger, and fighting tendencies. It is made of calcium carbonate and some chromium. It generally denotes Mars and blood.
4. Emerald - Green in color. It strengthens the nervous system and the communication of signals through the spine to the brain. It is made of beryllium silicate and represents mercury and the nervous system.
5. Yellow sapphire - Yellow in color. It increases luck, religion, blessings, and controls liver. It is made of silicate with abundant hydrogen element in it. It represents Jupiter and benefic
6. Diamond - white in color. It improves the reproductive belt, increases life comforts, attracts the opposite sex, art, movies, singing. It is made of carbon and represents Venus. It enhances pleasure.
7. Blue sapphire - blue in color. It increases bone strength, patience, capacity for hard work. It is made of iron and titanium with some zinc. It represents Saturn and balances ego.
8. Garnet - Deep red in color. It is made up of magnesium, calcium, aluminum, iron, manganese, chromium, but predominantly iron. It represents rahu the node, increases fear and helps to learn life lessons.
9. Cat's eye – multi-colored. Made of beryllium and

aluminum oxide. It makes sudden changes in life and helps to learn life lessons. It represents ketu the node

'There are some semi-precious stones which work somewhat like the original stone, but with lesser efficiency' said guruji. 'Aquamarine can replace emerald. To a smaller degree, Peridot can replace aquamarine. Similarly, opal can replace yellow sapphire to a smaller degree.'

'This body is a combination of carbon and hydrogen, as are all organic matter described in chemistry. Carbon, which is an Earthly element and hydrogen, which is an atmospheric element constitute the body. To that we add water, fire, and ether or space and the body is constituted. Ether is now considered a pathway as has been seen in the dark particle experiment conducted in Europe in 2019. This experiment gave humanity their greatest understanding of the black hole, yet. We shall dwell upon this topic a little later in our conversation. Let us, for the present, return to the subject of the stones. These stones, when set in a carrier metal like gold, silver, or platinum, carry the eddy current by creating a different magnetic pathway and goes to different glands depending upon the finger of the hand that you wear them on. Since wearing a stone has side effects, the choice of how it should be worn, the carrier metal, and the finger of the hand on which to wear it, should be left completely to the astrologer, who also should understand your wants.'

'This science of stones is a part of curative astrology devised to try and reduce the suffering of people and help them in at least partially achieving their wants. Under no circumstances does it ignore the purpose of life.

I asked Guruji, 'How these stones should be worn?'

Guruji replied, 'Normally these stones are worn as on rings on different fingers. The rings are cast in some carrier metal such as gold, silver, or platinum. The science of making you wear these stones on your fingers is that the nerves from different fingers are connected to the different glands, or electrical distribution points. So, the little finger is connected with the kidneys, adrenal gland, and nervous system and is considered for the water pipelines of the body. The ring finger is connected to the solar plexus and is concerned with the fire in the body. The middle finger is connected to the bones and is connected with space in the body. The index finger is connected to the liver and to the hydrogen element. Therefore, it is connected to movement. The thumb is connected with the reproductive organs and with the carbon element in the body.'

'If you are familiar with the science of acupressure or acupuncture, you will know that there are nerves in each finger that are connected to different glands as I just mentioned. These fingers carry the eddy current to those glands, thereby energizing them.'

'As far as astrology is concerned, both the fingers of the leg and hand are connected in a similar manner to these glands. But, for obvious reasons and practical purposes, you have to wear it on the hand.'

'Do some stones need a particular carrier metal, guruji?' asked Stella, who was particularly fond of platinum.

'Yes, Stella, that's right. Different stones need different carrier metals. For example, ruby, red coral, yellow sapphire, and emerald have to be cast in gold as the carrier. The carrier

metal for pearl is silver. And blue sapphire needs platinum as the carrier metal.'

'And, what about the right finger, guruji? How do we choose that?' I asked.

'You have to leave that to the astrologer, John. Only an astrologer can tell you that, depending on your wants.'

'Other than the atmospheric energies, there are also some energies related to the earth, which also influence people. The energies of this earth are magnetic, solar, and gravitational. This is another branch of science and you should have basic knowledge of this as well so as not to contradict the atmospheric energy. Solar energy runs from east to west, whereas magnetic energy represents north to south. The gravitational force is different at the equator as compared to the other latitudes. We should align our head and face north and east for most of the twenty-four hours of the day. Meditational and other activities for the uplifting of spiritual energy should be done as far away from equator, where the force of gravity is the lowest, as possible. This force is the lowest at the poles. This will not create conflicts specially if you have a disease and you are using atmospheric energies to cure them faster. The energies related to the earth are not as significant as the atmospheric energies or the science of stones.'

'As explained earlier, the stones act by changing your aura thereby creating different circumstances that support you. For example, one of the ways the circumstances could tilt in your favor is that you may get the support of other fellow human beings. Therefore, after wearing the stone in a ring, the person should observe even the tiniest change that may occur

that hints at whether the stone is giving you a better mindset to achieve your wants. If you do not observe these tiny changes, you may need to go back to the astrologer to explain what you experienced. Undoubtedly, stones will have some side effects and an astrologer is bound to inform you in advance and take your consent. Remember that to gain something you may have to lose something. Reflect on whether you are ready to absorb these small losses. Your choice of astrologer and faith on him or her is of utmost importance for guidance in life.'

'Besides curative astrology in stones, there are some hymns in every religion, which if chanted regularly and repeatedly, improve the secretions in glands. In Hindu astrology, each planet has a specific hymn, which have to be chanted in order to get the result.'

Guruji brought up a picture on the screen. 'This is an illustrative photograph taken by a kriyl camera for an aura of the body. When we have diseases, the aura connected with the chakra changes color and we become aware that the body has some disease in that portion. Similarly, when some curative methodology is used, we can spot the difference in the color of the aura within ten days to three months. This is one of the most significant evidences that can be produced in the science.'

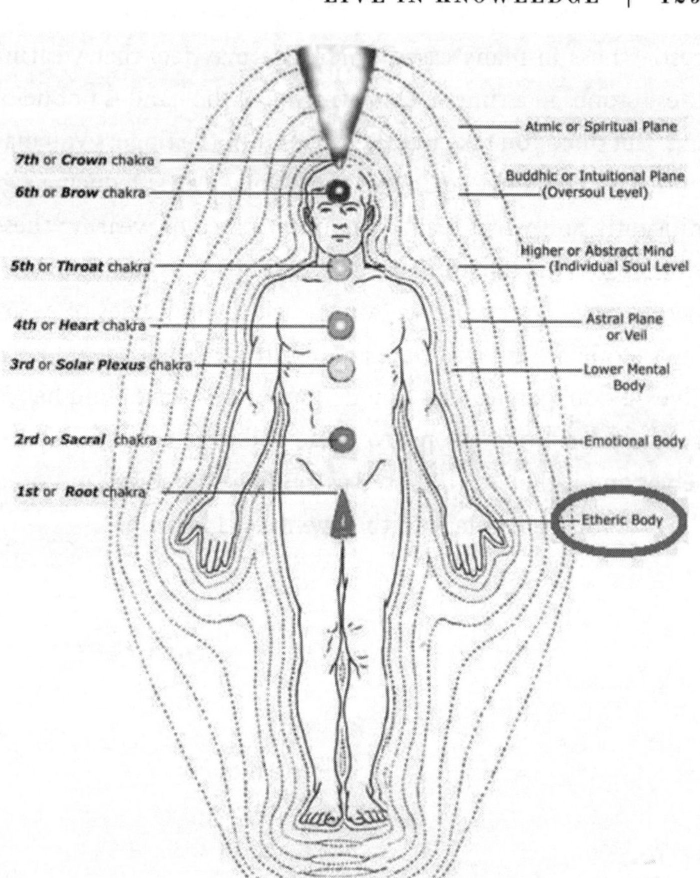

This is an illustrative photograph taken by a kriyl camera for an aura of the body
Sri Baheti

Guruji continued, 'But we must understand that these eddy currents can only take you half way to what you want to achieve. In the beginning, you are likely to see an immediate benefit, but then it reaches a saturation point beyond which you may not feel its impact significantly. This causes

restlessness in many cases, where we may feel that wearing these stones in a ring on some fingers of the hand is not helping. But once you take out the rings from the fingers you may notice that whatever gain had come your way is reducing significantly and you'll realize the importance of wearing these rings. 'Any way the proof of the pudding is in eating it, as they say. So one can try and see for oneself the efficacies of wearing a stone or several stones and figure out what advantage it gives. I don't advice that you do any of this on a blind belief. I would encourage people to come and test things for themselves and if they see themselves gaining something out of it, they can take advantage of the science as I believe.'

11

Success in Material World!

I was super excited to talk to Guruji the next day. I had spoken to the man whose journey into his past life I had witnessed on my trip to India. I had been able to confirm that guruji had been spot on in his analysis and was dying to let him know. As soon as we began, I said, 'Guruji, I spoke to the man who was hypnotized and had revealed secrets of his past life. I told him what you had predicted his axis of life. His life continues to be as sensational even now. Apparently, he earns reasonably well, but always wants more. And he is a gambler on the stock markets and continues to lose a significant amount of money there. He is desperately considering giving up this one habit that he blames for all his problems in life. He is also in trouble with the government as you had predicted, and I had confirmed.'

Guruji replied, 'Yes, but your excitement tells me that you have something more to reveal.'

'That's correct, guruji,' I replied. 'When I spoke to him

about what you had said about the village chief's axis of life, he was stunned. Apparently, one of his executives had always stood by him and helped him deal with the government cases. This former executive is a big shot himself, now, but continues to stay in touch with the man and helps him out as often as he can. Guruji, I am so excited that all your analysis on axis of life and theory of karma was so accurate in this case. However, it sends a chill down my spine to think that past life regression is possible and may even be important to know the axis of life and what we have to exhaust.'

Guruji replied, 'Well any knowledge that benefits human kind in some way is real knowledge. And what better goal can there be than to know the axis of life?'

After a pause, guruji continued "Life is the greatest adventure imaginable. Therefore, you should consider it a play and not take it too seriously. Very few lives have extra ordinary experiences. Otherwise, most lives are just mundane. Still people get depressed and end their lives, simply because they don't know how to play this game. My conversation with you, I hope, will prepare you to play it as casually as possible. I also acknowledge that material successes in this life means a lot and there is nothing wrong in desiring that or owning objects of comfort or luxury. But to make it the center piece of your focus will make you forget the real purpose of life. Therefore it is essential to keep a balance.'

'The main goal of most human beings is to be successful in this life. Their wants are also mostly the same. They all want a good personality, wealth, good house and property, good assistants, good education and children, a good spouse, good

luck, name and fame, steady source of income, and freedom from diseases and complications in life.'

'Well, these are the kind of things that only get fulfilled in fairytales, and sometimes not even in them. We have been born here to exhaust our elements. Unfortunately, no one normally remembers this until something happens in their life that sets them thinking as to the cause. The wants can be achieved partially or fully by utilization of energies and recharging or changing them by virtue of stones. But are worldly pleasures the source of happiness? The answer is clearly no. The purpose of this discourse is to navigate you through all the successes you achieve as well as the defeats that you encounter and learn what can be done when you face a defeat.'

'Let me tell you a story from Hindu mythology to illustrate my point.'

'It is said that we have three abodes, other than hell, which we can choose to visit after we die. The first one is heaven, where all kinds of pleasures, wealth, and all the good things of life are available. But the king of heaven, called Indra, is always insecure because he is constantly under attack from various evil beings and even rishis, or the scientists of yore, who, on the strength of their power, want to usurp the throne of heaven from Indra. Therefore, the king is always insecure. If you want a parallel from the modern world, think about how insecure some of the richest people in the world may be that they will be overtaken on that list by their rivals. They are probably always devising strategies for keeping these rivals at bay. This is true for all fields, such as sports or politics for example. Why, even countries have not been able to get over

such insecurities. Everything is a do or die battle for them, although all of them have plenty of pleasures already available to them.'

'Then we have the second abode of mount Kailash, where we have Shiva the eternal as the owner occupant. He does not need anything from this world and is happy living with his family on the top of that mountain in complete peace. Hunger and competition have no place on this mountain. Come to think of it, beings such as a lion, a bull, a peacock, a snake, and a mouse coexist in complete peace simply because they are each favored by different members of Shiva's family. However, there are very few takers for this abode of peace after death.'

'The last abode that we have is Vaikunth, where Lord Vishnu resides. This abode, which is in the middle of a vast ocean, is surrounded by beauty and prosperity because the goddess of wealth, Laxmi, is the consort of Vishnu. In this abode, there is no competition or hunger. As I described, it is opulent with prosperity and wealth. Hindus consider this as the abode that we should strive to achieve, because it is balanced. Therefore, balance in life is very important.'

'During challenging times, you need to rely on controlling the three bodies as explained earlier and try to surrender yourself to the all-powerful energy of which you are also a part and have some of it to make you sail through. The importance of this surrender is what we are emphasizing on in the present discussion. Life always does not go through the way you want it to. But, when you surrender, you experience peace and happiness and become in unison with the ultimate energy source. How do you surrender? There is no physical

surrender to anyone. You only surrender to yourself and the energy in you and the higher energy around you, thinking and wishing that they take care of you. That is what is called prayer. Prayer has a greater impact than all the other methods which I have suggested to you to achieve something. It starts with a humble request to the energy source and sometimes it takes or raises your will power to an extent that the universe is bound to give you a particular focused want.'

'Prayer combined with the willingness to accept any result the universe chooses to grant you is the best way. But, sometimes when your determination goes to the level of stubbornness and if what you desire is not in tandem with your axis of life, then you suffer. What I am now telling you is to pray positively for your wants at least three times of the day, clearly emphasizing your desire. But, then, leave it to the universal energy by surrendering to give you what it thinks best. You will see that more often than not, the universal energy will grant you what you seek. That is why you see all kind of boons granted to seekers, as described in the mythologies of different religions. That is how the universal energy surrenders to you sooner or later if you surrender with in depth, heartfelt prayer.'

Guruji continued, 'Once in a while, some good comes out of war also. It removes cowardice from within us. We should prepare ourselves for all kind of battles in this life. Hopefully, this discussion of ours will equip you with the weapons that you may need and also train you to be a disciplined soldier.'

However, there are times when we don't have an answer to the questions or challenges that life throws our way. So, how would you intuitively pick the correct path that you

must choose when faced with these challenges? Some psychiatrists advise us to sleep over the matter and let your subconscious decide the next day. However, I can suggest an exercise that can be done to help you arrive at a solution immediately. The first exercise is to rub your medulla oblongata. Most students of science might know that the medulla oblongata is a portion of the neck which joins the brain with the spinal column and all the nerves to the brain passes through this. As explained earlier, life gets into the body from this point through the pineal gland secretion. So it is a potent life force energizer point and massaging it creates the universal energy to respond to the challenge. If you want to look at it clinically, then you are simply improving the blood flow in this region, thereby supplying the mind with the fuel that it needs to think more intuitively.'

'Another exercise that is being recommended is to look at the open sky. You must sit or stand somewhere, where you can see the open sky and look at it as if you are seeing the universal energy. Wait for some time or do it couple of times without thoughts and with purity. You will experience a very strong idea coming into your mind and that will be the right decision to take to deal with the challenge. Again, if you want to look at this exercise scientifically, what we are doing is freeing the mental energy of all thoughts. Free from the shackles of thoughts, the mental energy is focused in space and the middle brain works better, combining to give you an answer. We must understand that all the answers lie within ourselves. Our mind, when connected to the universe, provides the best answers. The exercises are needed because they guide your subconscious in a manner that is beneficial to you.

They are recommended when you are in doubt as to what to choose. These are very serious exercises and you will have to have faith. Needless to say, you should have positive qualities in you to get the maximum benefit.'

I asked, 'Guruji, what greater challenge is there today than the virus that's spreading across the globe. Boston is also a hotspot now. Could we discuss diseases and how to cure them as that is the main focal point at present?'

'Certainly', said guruji, 'let us take this up tomorrow. However, it would be a good time to remember what Steve Jobs said before he died. That when things happen, you do not understand why it is happening to you. But when you look back from your death bed you realize that these dots were created specifically with a story for you and now when you join the dots you realize the meaning of it. So this COVID 19 may come and go one day and in some time in the future we will be able to join the dots to see why it come to us. So don't fear it the way you seem to be.'

I was wondering what my axis of life might be wouldn't it be great to know it and accept it and guide our life force in the right direction. It will avoid conflict with the universe at large and possibly make me successful in the material world. But will it be helpful in controlling any disease? Was my fear unjustified considering that the pandemic and its associated sad stories were all around?

12

Protection of Diseases Due to Acidic pH!

As soon as the call connected, I asked guruji, 'I understand that knowing the axis of life may help me achieve material success but how will it help in controlling diseases?'

Stella, who was probably fed up of my obsession with diseases, interjected before guruji could respond, 'Stress is what causes most body malfunctions. I think when the body is out of sync with the axis, it creates stress. I think that was what guruji was implying.'

Guruji joined the conversation, 'Yes, that's correct. In some practices, we suggest laughing as a possible solution to ward off stress. You simply laugh as loudly as possible and empty your mind of all stress. But there is more to the disease management than only stress management.'

I expressed my concerns to guruji, 'but, when we are only hearing sad and frightening stories of the pandemic every day, how can we be unaffected and without fear?'

Guruji replied in a calm voice, 'Once you know whatever

there is to know and start practicing it, you will not be affected by the sorrows of the world. Sorrows are the result of our attachments. If you practice all that I have described to you thus far, then all sad feelings will evaporate. Sad stories consist of matter vibrationary forces taking another shape. Take an example of ice. It is characterized by coldness, weight, and a form that we can see. When the same cube of ice melts, it becomes water. Pass electricity through this water and it divides into oxygen and hydrogen. It can no longer be seen but only felt. So look forward always and do whatever best you can keeping in mind all the conversations that we have had.'

'Like Stella said, fear creates stress and stress creates disease. Let me tell you a story to illustrate my point and also to show how we should deal with stress. Once upon a time a man with great magical powers used to live in a forest. Needless to say, such forests are teeming with wildlife of the most dangerous kinds in such stories. This person had a pet mouse that he really cared for. The mouse was very friendly and even visitors who came from afar to visit the man could not resist feeding it some tidbits. One day, a visitor came along bringing with him a cat. When the cat saw the mouse, all hell broke loose. A cat and mouse game of epic proportions ensued and finally the frightened mouse scampered on to the lap of its master for protection. Seeing his pet quaking with fear, the man was moved. Taking pity on the poor creature, the man invoked his magical powers and turned it into a cat. For a few days, things went on just fine. The mouse strutted around proudly, basking in the security of its new form. But, this was not to last long. One day, another visitor came along,

this time accompanied by a dog. The dog saw the cat and with a howl of pleasure pounced upon it. The cat was luckily very agile and with a screech of terror, landed on its master's lap once more. Once more, the master was moved by his pet's fears. Whether he ever considered putting up a board outside his ashram that animals were not allowed, I do not know. But he certainly did invoke his great powers and changed the cat to a dog. I guess when you have great magical powers, why should you bother with silly, practical ideas such as putting up notices!

Anyway, what was to follow could not have been prevented even if he had put up such a board. A hungry tiger happened to see this roly-poly dog bouncing about the ashram. Licking its chops with delight at the prospect of such an easy meal, the tiger bounded after the dog. With a yelp of terror, the dog leapt on to the lap of its master, its eternal source of refuge in times of danger. The man, who was used to having a tiny mouse leap on to his lap, was not prepared for the extra weight of the dog and was nearly knocked off his seat. Seeing what had caused his pet to take refuge in him, the man decided that he must put an end to the matter once and for all. Summoning his powers, he transformed the dog into a tiger. He also made a mental note to train his pet not to leap onto his lap any more.

The mouse turned tiger was bristling with pleasure at his new avatar. He had absolutely nothing to fear any more. On the contrary, he was now the source of fright for all the visitors who turned up at the ashram. Seeing this, the master would put his visitors at ease reminding them that the tiger was, after all, only a mouse and that they had nothing to fear

from it. The mouse-turned-tiger put up with it for a while, but then his tiger ego began hurting him. 'What!' he thought, 'this silly man thinks that I'm a mere mouse, does he? Then, I must teach him a lesson.' Thinking thus, the tiger turned to the man with a menacing growl. Seeing and recognizing the tiger's intentions, the master summoned his magical powers again and transformed the tiger back into a mouse.'

'The fear of diseases has become a monstrous tiger for us now. We need to change it back into the mouse that it really is. Let us not fear them unnecessarily, but identify the root causes of these diseases and take the necessary precautions.'

Guruji paused for a while to let us reflect upon his words. Then, he continued, 'None of us want diseases, but are we understanding what causes them? There are essentially two kinds of diseases. The first is caused by bacteria. In this category come diseases such as tuberculosis, typhoid, malaria, and dengue. These diseases can be mostly cured only through chemicals called antibiotics which we take as medicine so that the toxins of these bacteria are neutralized. In the good old days, when the allopathic system of modern medicine was not so advanced and such chemicals were not researched and available in the market, many people died due to diseases caused by bacteria. Thus, modern science has done a great service to mankind by keeping these diseases at bay and increasing the life expectancy of humans. Similarly the modern system has also done a great service by developing the ability to replace by surgery many worn out parts of the human body or even the chemicals accumulated within organs, such as kidney or gallbladder stones.'

'However, if you remember, I had suggested that the hu-

man being is capable of living until a hundred and twenty years of age. With all the advances in modern medicine, we have still not been able to achieve that. So, something is obviously missing. I have also suggested and explained earlier that the breath is a tool of enhancing life. The slower the breath the higher the expectancy of life, because the wear and tear of the body or cells depends upon the usage. So breath combined with modern science to take care of bacteria is certainly a way to prolong life. But the stress and strain of modern life is such that this breath control happens only some times of the day. It is not a constant occurrence. So, the our average reduction in breath per minute is very miniscule, although we can improve it by constantly being aware of it and following a disciplined life.'

'So how does modern life disturb us? One way is by making us run after material comforts. This requires a huge expenditure of energy of the mind. And are we satisfied with that? No. What we have must be better than what others have, because we are always competing with everyone that we know. This competition also utilizes a lot of energy. Then there are factors such as different time zones, different types of radiations that we are exposed to, the constantly agitated state of our mind, restlessness, the rapid pace at which things happen, and pressures imposed by our relationships. All of this affects the way the brain perceives threats and ultimately transfers it to different glands to act.'

'Once it comes under the purview of different glands, they become either hypo active or hyper active depending upon the signals emitted by the brain and we have all kind of diseases that either happen immediately or over some time. We

are not aware as to how to balance these chemical secretions from our glands and the first effect is that the toxic elements keep on getting accumulated more and more in the body.'

'I have explained earlier that the release of acids happens in the stomach due to increased activity in the brain. As a consequence, we over eat, to quench these acids. This is further compounded by the incorrect choice of food. So, the blood becomes more acidic and has more ash, or calcium compounds, or carbon dioxide as air bubbles in the arteries or some organs. This, ultimately, leads to diseases. I must add here that besides the choice of food, the way of eating is also very important. In our body, the biggest alkaline juice comes out of our saliva. So, the glands that produce saliva have to be healthy. The saliva should get mixed with the food to create a better PH balance when the food reaches the stomach after eating. Therefore, we must chew our food consciously and a lot more than we usually do to ensure that saliva is properly mixed in our food.'

'So the first way of prevention of diseases is to bring lifestyle changes. But, this is difficult to achieve. The second means of prevention is by avoiding choosing the wrong kinds of food. This is possible with some efforts. The third is to eliminate the accumulated calcium compounds and carbon dioxide, known as toxins in our body. The fourth is ensuring that these toxins are not deposited in some organs and arteries.'

'So we now know that the toxins are a major reason for diseases. In ayurveda, which is an ancient system of medicine that continues to be practiced in India to this day, it is understood that there are three types of diseases, other than bac-

terial diseases, caused by factors in the body. The first factor is kapha, which is fat or mucus. Then there is pitta, which is high acidity in the blood, which disturbs the pH level of the body. The third factor is vata or circulation of blood in different organs and arteries. All the non-bacterial diseases emanate from the misalignment of these factors. For a healthy body, it is essential to keep these factors in a proper proportion.'

'The kapha or fat or mucus is caused when metabolism is lower than what we eat. This creates more ash when the acid in stomach digests these foods and creates more calcium compounds by leaching excess calcium out of the bone marrow. It makes you obese and the mucus calcium compound gets deposited in various organs thus reducing their efficiency and giving rise to diseases.'

'The excess acidic blood causes organ failures and serious diseases including cancer. It is said that when the pH level of the body turns more acidic than the body can take, then the degeneration of tissues and muscles happen, again leading to diseases.'

The third reason is excess vata in the system, or in other words the obstruction of blood flow. This creates diminishing temperature difference between the temperature of the reproductive organs and the pineal gland. This could be due to a variety of reasons, including having an excess of carbon dioxide bubbles in the blood stream or constipation, resulting in the decreased evacuation of toxins from the body.'

'In general, if your intake of alkaline food is less or if there is a limited availability of alkaline minerals in the body to possibly clear the disturbance in the temperature gradient, then

the body becomes incapable or is limited in its ability to melt fat. This is known as the disease of the current or vata.'

So the diseases that occur in the body are due to one of the three conditions of kapha, pitta, or vata. These diseases are nonbacterial in nature and is thus in the second category of diseases which cannot be eliminated by using chemicals or antibiotic modern medicine.'

'Therefore, I recommend that these diseases be treated by different methodologies to get longevity. Modern medicine relies heavily on surgery to cure or change the diseased organ itself. This has its utilities, certainly. But, it diminishes the overall expectancy and feel of life.'

'I will explain in detail about some of these diseases subsequently where we will talk about diseases like cancer, pneumonia, or even the corona virus. We will see what they each are and what needs to be done when confronted by them. But, in general less of alkaline food intake or availability of less alkaline minerals in the body in disturbs the temperature gradient. The absence of the heat disrupts the melting of fat, which is accumulated in the body. Other problems are the creation of acidic blood due to carbon dioxide bubbles within the blood stream and constipation.'

'Therefore treatment on all the three bodies, like meditation for the causal body, controlling ego on the mental plane, and taking care of the physical body will yield wonderful results as far as health is concerned. Similarly, controlling these through astrology stones will also give a helping hand in taking control of a healthy life.'

'In this life, a normal human being looks for four types of pleasures. Health is right on top of this list. I will also de-

scribe the other general pleasures, which are not for the purpose of satisfaction of ego but generally increases the pleasure of life. So, the second pleasure that human beings seek in life is wealth. The third is having a meaningful spouse or partner because living alone in life is difficult. The fourth is having obedient children because they take care of you when you grow old and do not leave you at the mercy of caretakers at an old age home. Therefore, when you live life you concentrate on all these pleasures of life. Health, as I just described, comes right up on top. Other pleasures, such as properties and fame are all simply to feed the ego and making a statement to the world that even I am something significant.'

'We have discussed in detail how it is important for the organs of the body to be healthy for our overall health. We have also spoken of the significance of the temperature gradient between the reproductive organs and the pineal gland. The biggest contributors toward maintaining this temperature gradient are the bones of the body, which contain marrow. Marrow is a warehouse of all the alkaline metals of the body. If the stock of alkalinity in the marrow is enough or if we are consuming enough alkaline foods to maintain the temperature healthily in the reproductive organs, then the same will ensure that the mucus or toxins in the organs are melted from time to time so as to keep the organs healthy. The temperature can also be better maintained if the body's requirement of energy is less.

'How do we lower the requirement of energy in the body?' asked Stella

Guruji said "Most of us feel that if we rest the energy requirement of the body will be reduced. Moderate sleep does

so, but if you are lying down but not sleeping, then that may not be the case.'

Guruji said, 'Essentially, a lower breath rate requirement per minute and a stable and calm mind are also important in achieving this. If this is coupled with eating healthy alkaline foods of higher pH, then we can lead a healthy life without being afflicted by many diseases.'

'Let's once again examine the food that we eat. Obviously, meat and other non-vegetarian foods are highly acidic and not conducive to prolonging life beyond a certain age as explained earlier. And, food that is violet outside as well as inside is the most alkaline food which will prolong your life. In this category comes dragon fruit, which is violet colored inside and outside as well as violet-colored figs. There are very few violet-colored foods available, but these act directly on the pineal gland which controls the temperature gradient and maintains the temperature difference between the reproductive organs and the pineal gland.'

At this point, guruji brought up a picture on the screen. 'Take a look at this picture. You will observe that the colors go in a circle and the theory is that the violet color cures and pulls up all the colors in the VIBGYOR and thus improves the functions of these glands. Similarly, indigo will be able to cure all the glands of BGYOR, other than the violet color. And Thyroid with Blue color can help correct GYOR and so on. The red color pulls down the violet color most in a circular motion and thus reduces life. In this color theory we consider tomato to be the main red color which causes acidity and thus the temperature will be made higher at pineal gland level and thus reducing the temp difference essential to run the life. So

choice of food color wise is very important to maintain the temperature difference

While it is true that the color Violet pulls the indigo pituitary gland health most but it also to some smaller extent pulls up the glands below this as blue and to more smaller extent green and so on.

I therefore need to recommend even to eat the flowers which can be eaten with violet color or indigo color as some kind of made up food to really prolong life and keep organs healthy

I intervened" guruji do you see violet fish is better than other color fish?"

Guruji said" I think so though I have no practical knowledge of the benefits of violet color fish but the theory holds good"

"But there are other criteria's also of what we say specifically marked food for improving particular organs functioning "

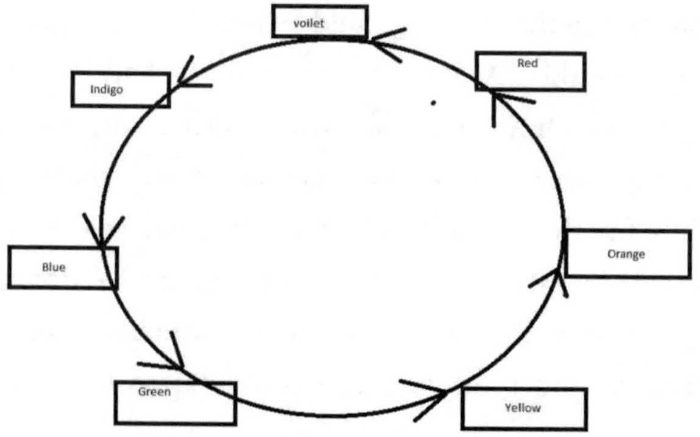

Guruji continued, 'Have you noticed that there is a similarity between some of the internal organs and external organs of our body? For example, the shape of our eyes is very similar to the shape of the liver. Similarly, the ears are shaped like the kidneys and our lips are shaped like our pancreas. So, if the lips aren't pink, or are cracked and chaffed, it is very likely that your pancreas need attention. There is an interesting test that you could do right now to see if your kidneys are in good shape. Try folding your ear till it touches the side of your head. If you find this difficult to do, then it could be an indication that there is some blockage in your kidneys. In fact, folding of the ears is a proactive exercise to keep your kidneys healthy. Similarly, keeping the eyes clear by regularly splashing it with cold water is a good way to keep the liver healthy. Redness in the eyes could be a sign of a heated fatty liver. As a corollary, a fatty liver could also cause cataract in the eyes.'

'We have already seen how nature has provided us with foods that are shaped like some of our internal organs and how consuming these foods could be beneficial for the organs that they resemble. As a quick revision, we had learned that the apple, which is heart-shaped, is great for the heart. Cashew nuts and red beans that are kidney-shaped work splendidly for the kidneys. The walnut is the shape of brain and apricots and dates resemble the reproductive organs. So, the lesson here is that there are several proactive things that you could do and food that you could eat to keep yourself healthy.'

These foods are normally high in alkaline content. So, they are essential to keep the diseases away. Equally impor-

tant is the evacuation of toxins to ensure that mucus, calcium compounds, and fat are not deposited in the body. One way to ensure that these deposits do not block the organs or arteries is to practice yoga.'

'Yogic exercises target specific organs and joints which are major spots where such compounds generally get deposited. I will not go into the details of these exercises, or asanas as they are known. Instead, I will recommend a couple of them that you could do every day. The first is called surya namaskar. Translated, it means 'salutations to the sun' or 'prayer to the sun'. But, it really is a very good form of physical exercise. This exercise will keep your spine in good shape and all the problems related to the distance between the D3 and D4 bones, pain, and slip disc will be minimized.'

'The second is called Kapal Bhati, which is a breathing pranayama exercise. This is done by pressing the region of the stomach below the naval and simultaneously pushing the anus up while drawing in the breath. The breath is then exhaled out effortlessly and naturally. This pull and push action clears the pathway for the temperature to travel up to the brain. However care should be taken that only the portion of the stomach below the navel is pulled. Also, obese people may find this difficult to achieve so it should be slowly built. If too much pressure is exerted, it can exert pressure on the heart. So, great care needs to be taken and this exercise should be done gently. The breathing exercises, or pranayama as they are called, involve the drawing in of a deep breath by the means of the stomach and the lungs. This breath is held for as long as possible while pulling in the anus and then releasing the same. This exercise alone is called jalandhar bandh which

means packing the breath in the stomach and chest area and ensuring that oxygen reaches each and every cell of the body. This exercise alone is capable of making the lungs healthy and keeping viruses like COVID and illnesses like pneumonia away. You can get more details on this asana from Google or other sources. But doing these exercises regularly will give you a better chance of proactively warding off diseases. In yoga, you have specific exercises for all kinds of orthopedic pain of different joints and even exercises of the brain to prevent conditions like Alzheimer's.

'Basically, these exercises create a better blood flow towards the area to which they are directed. This helps to remove mucus, fat, or calcium by filtering them out through the kidneys. There are other methods also to improve the blood flow and primary among them is massage.'

'The massage that I speak of is not the general massage that we may be able to experience in a spa. These are massages that are directed to each and every organ. You may not find these in great detail on Google or other sources, so I will now describe a few of them.'

'You could do a massage that is beneficial to the brain by simply gripping the hair on your head and pulling and holding it for ten seconds. Do this four or five times ensuring that you cover the scalp in its entirety. This will ensure that clots are not formed anywhere in the brain.'

'You could also massage your head. To do this, press the corpal side of your head and the center of the head near the eyebrows for 20 seconds with your fingers. Massage the medulla oblongata for half a minute so as to avoid spondylitis

and release any tension that is built up due to anxieties and responsibilities.'

'You can also massage the top and bottom of your lips. For this, place a finger of one hand horizontally over the upper lip and a finger of the other hand below the lower lip. Press the two fingers in opposite directions to massage the lips.'

'As you have learned, saliva is a very important enzyme that contributes to the alkalinity and digestion of food. As the body ages, saliva generation decreases. A good way to ensure that the saliva flow is maintained is to exercise the salivary glands by pressing the jaw toward the ears using the thumb and index finger of both hands.'

'To massage the thyroid gland, press the throat pipe gently with thumb and index finger and slide it down to the base of the throat.'

'You could also get a deep tissue massage of your chest, stomach, back, and leg muscles massaged at a spa to clear the deposits along the bones.'

'There are two specialized massage that you have to do yourself. The first is the massage of the tail bone so that deposits do not pile up there. If this happens there is the danger of the tail bone expanding and blocking the temperature transfer upward toward the brain. If deposits are allowed to accumulate at the tail bone over a period of time, then they become hard like a bone. Doctors then recommend that this be removed surgically.'

'Another area that you need to massage is your pelvic area and genitals. The area between the anus and the genitals is a hot spot for maintaining the temperature and needs to be massaged. It is also close to the urinary bladder, which is a

potential location for infections as the body ages. This massage is thus helpful for the overall health of the body. The pelvic area deep massage also takes care of prostate and ovarian cancers. The massage of the genitals is necessary to keep the blood flow into those areas and not make them a dead muscle.'

'You may not possibly be able to imagine the advantages of this massage at your age. But believe me, your old age will be much better if you do these massages and not allow the muscles to become dead by virtue of stopped blood flow.'

'This entire process of yoga and massage will not take more than 15 minutes of your daily life. But, it will help you save millions when you are old. It is also true that when the physical body is healthy, you can have better spiritual or mental plane exercises as explained in our earlier discussions, thus exhausting the elements for which you were born.'

'What we have discussed thus far today are proactive ways to keep diseases away. We have not spoken of any prevalent medical beliefs to fight diseases. I have described earlier that bacterial diseases are best controlled by taking modern medicine chemicals and antibiotics. Modern medicine often takes the route of surgery to treat diseases of the body organs. However, these procedures are accompanied by pain and side effects. There are other alternative medicines that also need to be considered. Homeopathy, which originated in Europe, deals with working on the body's immunity through the patient's mind. The Tibetan medicine works through various herbs found in the Tibetan region. India's own ayurvedic herbal treatment which I spoke of briefly earlier is another branch of medicine as is the Chinese traditional methodol-

ogy. All of these have their advantages. It all depends upon the faith of an individual. But there are success stories in these as well and I will certainly recommend trying them for general upkeep.'

Stella said 'Guruji, the biggest killer among all modern diseases is cancer. I think every tenth woman that I know has either breast cancer or cancer of the ovaries or uterus. Can the treatment methods that you described to us help with cancer, too?'

Guruji replied, 'Definitely, since the steps will help improve general health, it will also have a positive effect on preventing cancer. But let me talk to you about cancer as well as COVID tomorrow. Hopefully, you will the understand why these happen and what is the best that we can do to reduce their chances.'

Stella summarized that "we now understand food which causes acidic blood but are there any other reasons?"

Guruji said, "The biggest reason for acidic blood is continuous thinking and thoughts in the mind, that is why I have stressed about meditation and all other habits described beforehand."

" If we can nip the source in time that is at a young age we can really protect us from the big trouble which can happen once we get little old" Guruji said

14

Knowledge about Cancer!

Guruji said, 'Most people are frightened at the mere mention of the word cancer. It is certainly the one disease of modern times that takes the greatest toll in terms of human life. So, let's now talk about how cancer is caused and how it can be prevented or cured.'

'In the past, human life expectancy was lower than what it is today. So, cancer, which usually happens in old age, was more or less unheard of. People back then used to die of bacterial diseases and the average life expectancy was around fifty years. Cancer usually afflicts people over the age of fifty, though there are definitely cases of people much younger than that contracting the disease. Cancer can also be considered to be a modern day disease because of modern lifestyles and beliefs. I have discussed earlier that diseases other than bacterial diseases are formed because of obstructed blood flow and because of a greater acidic pH of the blood. While both of these are causes of death, the acidic pH is a primary

cause. Because of our poor habits and life stresses, about which I have tried to educate you in detail via our earlier discussions, the blood starts becoming acidic after a certain age.'

'The blood flow was also used differently, earlier. You may wonder how blood flow can be used! Here's an example. In the past, women used to have more children and breast milk was fed to the children for a considerably longer period of time. This is true universally, not just in some third world countries. Even in the United States, women had, on average, more children than they do now. So, back then, the flow of blood to the breast could be naturally handled. But now, with lesser number of children and a tendency to minimize the use of breast milk, the milk and its components, which are generally acidic, form lumps in the breast and that is the biggest cause of breast cancer. Having fewer numbers of children is also the cause for cancer of the uterus. The uterus is not used as much as it was when women bore many children and this has reduced the blood flow to this organ, causing ovarian and uterus cancer. One way to reduce the occurrence of these cancers is to make use of the massages we spoke about last time.'

'Now, let us examine what happens with more acidic blood. The acidic blood attracts the body fat or kapha cells and forms a layer engulfing the acid on top of an organ. Over time, the layer of kapha with acid contained becomes thicker and thicker and does not allow the organ to continue its function. If the acidic blood continues in the body, this excess of kapha attraction also happens in other organs and we then call it metastasis of cancer, which means that the cancer has spread to other areas as well. But the basic cause of all these

problems is acidic blood. Mind you, it is impossible to turn acidic blood back into an alkaline nature in a short period of time. Therefore, it is very difficult to find a cure. I have a cure in mind which is semi-surgical in nature and needs to be supplemented with the intake of alkaline foods. But this has never been tried in a clinical research as yet and that is why I cannot speak of it now. Maybe, with god's grace, a research agency may be interested in exploring this idea. Then I can certainly try to contribute to the research on this disease that the best scientists in the world are indulging in.'

'We have spoken in detail about some of the alkaline foods. One that I had briefly touched upon is "ghee" or clarified butter extracted from the milk of "Gir" cows. Gir cows are found in some parts of India and the ghee extracted from their milk is very alkaline.'

Guruji took another pause.

Suddenly, my phone started ringing. It was my friend, Dennis Blue, who was on a cruise somewhere in the Atlantic. I excused myself for a second and answered the call. Dennis was sounding a little worried. Apparently, some people on-board the ship had tested positive for the virus and no country was allowing the ship to dock.

After trying our best to reassure Dennis, Stella told him, 'Dennis, we are in discussion with our Indian mystic Guru about knowledge which can be acquired to help us lead a happy life. We are on the chapter of cancer and are talking about how it originates and what can be done to control it. We are also surely going to discuss the corona virus situation with him. So why don't you join via conference call later when we are on corona subject?' Dennis replied that his

mother-in-law who was also on the cruise with him was suffering from cancer and so was curious to know what we had discussed on cancer thus far.

We requested guruji to give some knowledge to Dennis as well. Guruji replied, 'There were certain medicines which possibly can be given to patients on the high seas of the Atlantic, but cannot be prescribed in the USA as they are not approved by the FDA both for cancer and corona virus. So I cannot prescribe them as well. However, these medicines are practiced in India and some of the European countries as well.'

'Some of these are astrological medicines, which can be made from the same stones that are recommended for wearing. These medicines are made by oxidizing the stones and making them work internally by directly acting on the appropriate glands, thereby increasing life span. These are all approved by the Indian Ayurvedic system though some modern doctors object to these due to presence of metals in them. Whether they cause problems to the system or the kidneys is a view that is being hotly debated these days. So, these medicines may not be available in the US, though they are in India.'

'But there is no dispute about alkaline food. So, this is an aspect that must be understood very clearly by all.'

'There is another type of cancer which is myeloma, or blood cancer. This is different than other types of cancer. In this, the acid in the blood draws more minerals from the bone and marrow to produce more energy. But the minerals are not replenished and eventually the body's mineral stocks get depleted. The bones become hollow and the marrow does not

carry enough minerals. That's when myeloma sets in, requiring a marrow transplant. So wisdom lies in controlling the acid by keeping your mind stress free and in a happy state, and mostly eating alkaline food. I have spoken earlier about what and how you can do that on the spiritual and mental plane to reduce stress. Please understand that thoughts are indestructible. So, even though you may not speak out or verbally express angry thoughts to avoid confrontations, they still cause stress and then create acidity. This acidity, over a period of time as explained above, can cause cancer. For the patient on the Atlantic Ocean cruise, I would like to recommend an Indian herbal drug, which is called soot sekhar ras, for handling this though I doubt you can find it on board. However, this drug is a combination of mercury and sulfur, two ingredients not liked and therefore banned in the US. If you recall our discussion on the reason for birth, you may remember that it is because of the interaction of sulfur and mercury as the sperm and the egg. So, consuming a compound of mercury and sulfur should be researched before it can be prescribed. Undoubtedly over the years and with age the capacity of the kidneys to flush out mercury diminishes and that becomes a valid reason for concern. But a sporadic usage to control the pH of blood is still recommended in India.'

'Other addictive habits that increase acid formation is the consumption of alcohol and smoking. These are two habits that you may want to quit entirely or at least moderate.'

'Constipation can also cause cancer of the colon. This happens when the evacuation process is slow, resulting in some constipation. Acidic blood compounds the whole effect.

Therefore it is important to maintain body functions as I explained earlier to ward off the evil of cancer from our life.'

I reflected upon all that guruji had said. 'Guruji, it is true that cancer is something that scares people very much. But it progresses slowly and gives us a couple of years to live. In many cases, people have gotten out of it also if it was detected in time. But COVID 19 gives us no time. So please let us hear your views on COVID 19.'

'Let's do that tomorrow, John', said guruji, looking at his watch. So, we scheduled the most important discussion in the present context to the next day. Dennis also wanted to join on the discussion about corona and he was advised the timing of the call.

As had become our practice, Stella and I spoke for some time after the meeting about the things that we had discussed. We wondered what the possible remedy for cancer that guruji had hinted upon was. Would some research agency be willing to consider it? Perhaps, some agency would in the future and the world may have another chance of getting rid of one of its biggest killers.

15

COVID Knowledge and Control!

'The entire world is now in the grips of panic due to a virus. It is not like there have not been similar viruses before. We have had H1N1 and Ebola epidemics across the world as well. However, none of those epidemics have captured the imagination of the world like this one has. Apart from the phenomenal numbers of people that this disease has claimed, it is understood that the pneumonia that happens as a result of COVID 19 infection causes a great deal of discomfort. This disease is new and none of the big research labs have done much research on this phenomenon. But what I am going to say may shed some light on the cause or reasons for this disease and likely suggest a cure, though this has not been clinically tested on many human subjects as yet.'

'This disease is also a product of the excess acidic nature of the blood, which is why it seems to affect the elderly more. In this case the acid in the blood gets a mucus deposit in the tissues, interacting with the proteins in the muscles due to

cold air passing through the nostrils, eyes, or ears. In some cases, the head's exposure to cold also creates the protein to stick to the acid. Since this disease is due to cold air or waves passing through the nose, ears, eyes, or head the first place which the air hits is the throat. The excess acid in the blood, along with the protein, creates a virus layer. When this layer is exposed to cold air it gets stuck in the tissues. The acidic blood also continues to wreak havoc on the tissues. Having an reflux problem and being on some antacid alone does not make less acidic blood. Over time, the layer of acid and protein finds its way to the lungs .If more acid is available in the stomach the acid reflux happens up to the throat then there is a possibility that the liquid may cross over from the food pipe into the wind pipe. From there it might enter the lungs and cause pneumonia. It might interest you to know that the only difference between this disease and earlier diseases of a similar nature is that COVID 19 is a disease of fusion.'

'Fusion! I exclaimed, nearly jumping out of my chair in excitement, 'fusion with what?'

Guruji said, 'Calm down, John. Restlessness of any nature is not good. I do appreciate your inquisitive nature, though. The fusion that I am talking of is between a bacterial disease and a non-bacterial disease. Essentially, the disease has traces of malaria or similar such poison in it, possibly due to the nature of its origin. Sometimes small traces of poison remain in the body due to insects bite or consumed food or even with a past malarial history of the patient. When this toxin gets combined with the acid blood and mucus deposits, it creates a very firm grip on the organs of the body. Therefore no single treatment is effective as such and we need to have a chem-

ical compound to treat the bacterial mix, while at the same time treating the non-bacterial side of the disease. The solution is to build immunity and also use the steam inhalation to break the cold air which fuses the entire virus effectively. Besides this we have to take care that the acid reflux could cause pneumonia as we discussed just now. So, it should be controlled fast. The malarial poison always has a tendency to travel to the brain fast. So, care has to be taken there as well.'

So in both situations, where you are either taking antacids regularly or are suffering from acid reflux there is a danger of COVID during winter time.

'Younger persons who have been affected also have acidic blood pH. Therefore, a diet composed predominantly of alkaline food and limited or controlled exposure to cold air will be a good precaution. I'm aware that "cold" is a relative term. What is cold for us in India may not be cold for you in the US. Also recall the discussion we had on the temperature gradient within everyone. People who have an optimum temperature gradient within them are able to withstand COVID more effectively because their immunity is better.'

'The fact that COVID 19 is a fast progressing disease can also be used to control it. Unlike cancer, which spreads slowly, COVID 19 can be acquired by anyone who is exposed to the virus because all people have some acidic pH in their blood. But the advantage is that it can also be cured faster than cancer and by employing much simpler methods. Unlike cancer, COVID does not create layers after layers of fat or mucus. However, complications such as pneumonia can make it deadlier too.

'So what is the cure for COVID? None of the techniques

or methods that I'm going to describe have been put thorough clinical trials, mind you. But these are simple exercises that we have already described in our earlier discussions. For example, let us control our exposure to cold air, which is the binding factor. Steam inhalation is a good way to loosen the binding. Let us drink warm water instead of room temperature or cold water. Avoid using ice in your drinks. Perhaps it is a good time to remind you to avoid alcohol consumption altogether. But that may be easier said than done. So, let us try to limit it as much as we can and avoid ice altogether. Practice pranayama or the breathing exercise that I described earlier. In order to prevent the acid and protein combination from slipping into the lungs, sleep on your stomach at night, even if you have dry cough. Keep on taking longer and deeper breaths as often as possible every day.'

'Besides this we need to eat foods that are considered "hot" in nature to be able to dissolve the mucus compound on the acid. What are these "hot" or "heat generating" foods? Turmeric, black pepper, cinnamon, cloves, big cardamom, and onions are all spices which are heat-generating. Consuming these will create heat and melt the mucus stuck on the acid. Once the mucus is melted the acid gets dissolved in the blood. To clear the acid from the blood, you could use the techniques I explained in our earlier discussions.'

'Besides this you can take a neem giloy, known in English as tinospora cardifolia tablets or drink a tea made by heating the bark of the tree itself. Then we have a powder of spices such as saunth (Zingiber officinale), black pepper, peepal (piper longum), laung (cloves), chhoti elaichi (Elettaria cardamomum), badi elaichi (ammomum subutalum), jayphal,

javitri (Myristica fragrans), cinnamon, tulsi or basil (ocimum sanctum), which when taken with warm water is very curative. In order to increase immunity you have to rely on shilajit or mineral pitch in English along with shranga bhasma (made out of deer horn). These are Indian ayurvedic medicines and they are permitted to the best of my knowledge in the US as well.'

Since Dennis was on SOS, Guruji asked him to drink only warm water and try steam inhalation at least a couple of times in the day. He was also advised to sleep on his stomach. If he was able to find some cloves, black pepper, cinnamon, and honey in the kitchen he would have a home remedy on his hands. He was to suck the cloves till they dissolved, and not chew them. The rest of the ingredients he was to mix to a paste and consume three times a day to ward off any potential problems.

'Homeopathy also recommends using Camphor 1 M and arsenic album 30 as two medicines for helping fight the virus by creating antibodies in your body. This is similar to giving plasma of a person who has been cured of Corona to a patient to allow the patient's body to develop anti bodies.'

'Unfortunately the research is not taking into account how this virus occurs. And since the clinical suggestions are less expensive they are not a toast of big research firms. What modern medicine is trying to do by introducing the plasma of a recovered patient into a patient suffering from the virus is certainly a cure. But, since this virus can keep coming again and again over time, a cheaper and more effective cure is most desirable.'

'I have told you what you could do to specifically deal with

this disease. Please understand that the disease itself is not as deadly as our ignorance is making it seem. If you faith in my advice, then please convey these measures to more people so that we may be able to contain this disease fast.'

I asked, 'Guruji, so why is the world not trying these cures? Do they have any side effects?'

Guruji replied, 'Most herbal and homeopathic medicines do not have side effects. But I am not aware as to what the legal processes are before these can be tried in your markets. Otherwise, I could have ensured their availability in your market for trial with patients.'

Guruji further continued, 'The problems that we face in this world are actually not too big, but we blow them out of proportion. We could cut them to size by simply living the way our ancestors did for so many years of human existence. Instead, we choose to rely on an incomplete science that we learned in school. No one wants to make life simpler as this does not serve the interest of the big lobbies that control the health care industry. Let us leave it at that.'

'Do we need to discuss any other types of diseases, guruji?' I asked.

'We do, John', he replied, 'but since we have addressed one of your biggest concerns today, I will leave you to reflect upon that. Let us pick up our discussion tomorrow.'

Stella and I spoke about all that we had learned about COVID 19 that day and what we could do to keep us away from the dreaded disease and its fear.

The techniques that were discussed were so simple that I could not think of what harm they could ever cause. Steam inhalation to break the cold air which helps breaking the

chain, was such a simple thing to do. Anyone who had a tea kettle and a small pipe could do it effectively. That got me wondering why ventilator manufacturers could not think about heating the oxygen which is delivered to a serious patient on this support system. What side effects could that possibly have?

I also did not have answers for the why homeopathic and ayurvedic drugs were not being put on trial, even though these did not have any side effects. Perhaps they could be tried on patients with milder symptoms to begin with to test their efficacy. But the world was what it was and though this pandemic had given the world a chance to reboot, I doubted if any of these apparently sensible options would even be considered.

However I also remembered that guruji had said that we must first be the change that we wanted to see in the world. Therefore, I decided to follow Guruji's instructions on this.

16

Protection from Disease of Fat/Kapha!

Guruji said 'Let me talk to you some other kind of diseases which are primarily caused by Kapha or mucus or fat or calcium compounds.'

'We have seen the nonbacterial diseases caused by the acid blood. The other kinds of diseases are caused by the ash, calcium compound, mucus deposits on organs and arteries. This creates a situation where the organ cannot function at its normal efficiency. So, the organ becomes diseased and has to be replaced by surgery according to modern science. There are cases where stones are formed of calcium compounds in the gall bladder or kidney and they have to be surgically removed. Sometimes the blood itself becomes thicker and slows down its flow or clots form to slow the flow further. To treat these conditions, you are then advised to use blood thinners, or reduce your blood pressure, or use clot-dissolving medicines to rectify the problems.'

There are some natural blood-thinning foods, such as

pomegranates, but even they are incapable of dissolving mucus. They also do not dissolve mucus. The mucus is best dissolved by eating heat-producing food that we spoke about yesterday. Here's a quick recap of some of these foods - turmeric, black pepper, cinnamon and so on. It is always advisable to consume these spices regularly. Massages are also beneficial in clearing mucus by dissolving it in the blood. Some kinds of acupunctures also help in clearing these by sending some low currents through the pathway. Other remedies are to follow yogic exercises.'

One of the things that help you manage these is taking detox medicines, which are essentially laxatives, to excrete these compounds from the body regularly and at a faster rate. Another way is to fast for at least four days in a month. Some religions have fasting built into their religious rituals, simply because of the many benefits of this phenomenon. Remember that the body's energy requirement decreases with age. So, adjustments in food habits and in the quantity of food consumed are required. Most of modern day dieticians give importance to this aspect and are thus credible. However the only caution to be exercised is to make sure that you do not underfeed yourself. The energy requirement of the brain is dependent on the nature of your work. If you underfeed yourself, you could increase the acidic blood in your system and will thus get caught in the other kind of diseases or disorder. So a balance of everything must be achieved according to your individual requirements. Exercising care is of utmost importance because while we are taking care of one issue, we may be inadvertently slipping into others.'

'The other kind of disease is the accumulation of bubbles

of carbon dioxide in the blood. This, as we have discussed earlier, restricts the flow of blood to the organs where the carbon dioxide is allowed to accumulate. These, as we have learned earlier, are called vata diseases. They create major pains in the joints, sciatica, rheumatism, and spinal cord disorders because the transmission of blood is reduced. The only way out is the use of purgatives, so that these bubbles pass out of the body in the natural course. Another thing to be cautious about is not to have too much of acidic foods if we also have a mucus constitution as a natural composition of our body. If we do and we consume too many foods that are acidic in nature, this will create carbon dioxide. Conversely, if we have more acid blood, we should take care not to eat food that is difficult to digest as this will also create excess of carbon dioxide.'

'If we take all these precautions, we can definitely live to the age of a hundred and twenty without diseases. Remember what we said about organ replacement. Modern science may be able to replace diseased organs and joints in the body, but it cannot ever give the same sense of fulfillment or expectancy of life that the organs that we are born with can provide. Living a long life is a dream of all human beings and no one wants to die at any age. Therefore living longer with happiness and joy should be our goal in life and the happiness and joy quotient should be increased by controlling the mental and spiritual planes as described earlier.

Stella again summarized" as apart from food what else can we do to let mucus or fat not accumulate in our body?"

Guruji said "Fat production happens when your metabolism rate is slower and that happens with you not adjusting to

your requirement of energy with age. However, besides this not doing yogic exercises so as not to allow accumulation of this produced fat is one definitive reason for fat to get deposited somewhere. Therefore the pranayama increases metabolism and different yoga postures exercise, if done regularly, insures that fat does not get accumulated inside the body. In fact modern science gives so much importance to do some kind of exercise every day. Yoga is only targeted exercise for different organs but regular exercise from swimming to cycling to plain simple jog or walking all helps. I have also explained that acid and fat combination becomes cancerous so special attention should be done to burn fat"

17

Protection of Diseases Arising of Current Flow!

Stella asked, 'Guruji, my friend has been diagnosed with auto immune diseases and she also suffers from rheumatoid arthritis. It is very crippling and painful. Are these auto immune diseases different then what you have mentioned.'

Guruji answered, 'Well most of the other diseases are derivative diseases of the main problems that I have narrated previously and they manifest in a person according to the weakest link broken in a chain. So these auto immune diseases, like rheumatism, are essentially a combination of mental plane and physical plane problems. But you are right about the fact that by the time we become aware of them, even the knowledge that I have shared is not enough to cure them immediately. The knowledge which I shared with you is not a medicine. But if we know it and practice it then we will improve health in a normal way including for rheumatism. But

in the short term, the medicines used in ayurveda are gold bhasma or oxidized gold. However, these medicines cannot be obtained in the US because they contain metals. It is interesting to note that modern medical science has a similar treatment of taking a course of gold injections for this condition. In homeopathy, you can use flower medicines as prescribed by Dr. Edward Buch, which cures the condition by changing your mental thought process. These are long lasting and without much side effects. But, do you know that meditation alone can also control this disease and can create a protective shield around us so that we do not suffer from these conditions.'

'I can see people suffering from arthritis, back ache and spondylitis. These are all debilitating diseases but the main reason for all of these is anxiety, load of responsibilities and financial problems that a person may be having. So the real cure is on the planes that I had shared with you earlier though some yoga exercises can also help in the short term. The outlook of a person is the causative factor of all such diseases and we must understand this.'

I asked, 'Guruji, what about diabetes, kidney ailments, and liver diseases? What can we do for these conditions?'

Guruji said, "Well, if you follow whatever I have shared with you so far, it can be beneficial in dealing with these diseases as well. If you already have these diseases, you can resort to modern medicines. For liver, including fatty liver, I recommend homeopathic medicine of natrum sulph 6X and cheladonium 200 and ayurvedic medicine of Punarnava. But, I would still advice you to start following whatever I have shared with you and you should start seeing results soon.'

'For diabetes and for help with the pancreas you must consume a good amount of curcumin, the source of which is turmeric. These are also diseases of the thought process.'

'For the kidneys, it would do well to remember that the element is fear. So, unless someone shares their lifestyle with me, I would be unable to suggest any medicines for immediate relief. But, yes, yogic exercises and massages will help in controlling it.'

'It would not be fair for me to suggest medicines if someone is diseased. So my advice should be considered only as a guiding tool to improve immunities as I am not a qualified medical doctor.'

I asked Guruji, 'How did you acquire all this knowledge?'

Guruji answered, 'I did not acquire any of this knowledge. It manifested itself in my subconscious by the grace of my guru and I narrated it for the benefit of the world at large after weighing it with the scientific knowledge that I received as a part of my education. I have always believed that the proof of the pudding is in eating it. So I tried these methods and my experiences have been good.'

'What about HIV?' I asked Guruji

'Well HIV is also an auto immune disease, which comes from the family of vata in ayurveda. Vata, as I explained earlier, is the blockage of blood flow due to air bubbles in the blood stream and heavy clots.

'Ayurveda describes a variety of activities by the means of which the gas in the blood stream can be released. Massage is an external activity. The use of laxatives can also help to clear the bubbles as much as possible. In India, we use herbal laxatives instead of the chemicals recommended by modern

medicine. The herbal medicine does have an advantage that it does not make the intestine and colon dry. The food for this is amla known as gooseberry. The herb is haritaki, called terminia chebula, which is a laxative used in ayurveda. The astrological medicine for this is to improve the carbon element in the body. So, Hirak Bhasma, which is oxidized carbon, is prescribed. Again, this can only be obtained in India and cannot be procured in the US. So, I will not advice it and possibly more research is needed.'

'The carbon element is an essential constituent of the CH combination from which all matter is made. So, it would be fairly easy to understand the importance of carbon.'

Stella summarized "that what you emphasize is that we should concentrate on elimination of toxins for keeping ourselves safe from the diseases born out of current flow"

Guruji said, "Yes we have elimination done through excretions through colon, through kidneys, and also through perspiration. All are important. We should observe these flows regularly and make sure that we are not deficient anywhere".

18

Living Longer!

I said, 'Guruji, you have given us so much knowledge about the specific disease COVID 19 which has caused so much havoc around the out the world. You have also spoken to us about Cancer, the most dreaded of killers in the modern world. I have no doubts that the world will benefit, sooner or later, from your immense knowledge. Do you want to say anything more to us?'

Guruji said, 'Like we have discussed so often in the course of our series of talks, the ancient scientists, or rishis, of India would live beyond the age of a hundred and twenty years. One of the most important of their practices was the way they moved from a frugal diet of fruits to living only on air. These rishis would only draw in very few breaths and concentrate heavily on their inner spiritual eye. Their faces radiated pure joy. I do not know how this can be achieved, but it is an ambition of mine to be able to discover some of their secrets if I can.'

Guruji further said, 'I am giving you some hints about some other methods to prolong life other than the ones that

I have already described. One of the things that mankind has yet to discover is how to use inert gases to cure diseases and prolong life. As explained earlier, life began by utilizing energy to bifurcate inert gases and thus causing the atom to separate into protons and electrons. The protons developed into alkaline substances and became sperms and the electrons remained as acidic substances and became acidic eggs.'

'Inert gases are presently not deployed as they are not soluble. They don't react because they have eight electrons in their outer atomic shell structure.'

'More research has to be done so that the electrons of this shell can be used to cure the condition of excess acid blood in human beings. At present, scientists agree that the inert gases have the power to create new tissues but they have not been able to find a way to do it. Once you find how to do this, then immortality or no death will be not a mere ambition with the human being but an actual achievement.'

'We are all aware that the human body is made out of atoms which vibrate at a certain frequency every moment. When these vibrations slow down, we need to recharge them with electrons of higher vibrations.'

'Here is an excerpt on how inert gases, which vibrate at a much higher frequency then the human atoms, behave. The scientists accept that all matter, including the matter that our human body is made of, consists of atoms that vibrate at a certain frequency, thus giving the shape of the matter. When this frequency becomes slower and slower, it results in diseases and death.

Inert-gas therapy is based on a concept that space is something, not nothing, as most scientists believe. This something

is called ether, which permeates all of our three and also higher dimensional space. A lot of research is needed to see how to make these inert gases work for repairing our bodies. Though some inert gas emitting devices are available in the market, their efficacy is not known. In my view, the inert gases have to be made to shed some electrons to the human cells and therefore have to be soluble in blood. But for your knowledge I am describing the inert gas device as claimed by the manufacturer and submitting their science and their mechanism.'

At this point, guruji brought up a part of an article on the screen.

'The actual mechanism and explanation for the resulting PE (Primary Energy) ray emitted from an inert gas device is that the magnetic field excites the inert gas atom (AKA *excitation*) to such a vibration that it "unmasks" the aether. In the late 19th century and early 20th, it was postulated that the aether is the space between all things and its behavior was more like fluid as opposed to the nothing which for most of the 20th century it was thought to be. Recent advances in physics with string theory and quantum physics now allow physicists to speculate that the space between all things, also known as "dark matter" does behave very much like a fluid, although it is not composed of infinitely small particles as once postulated pre Einstein. In the experiments using the LHC (Large Hadron Collider) these theories may be proven and a whole new world of physics will open to the scientific community with the observations made on dark matter and

dark energy. To further understand this theory, let's look at Dark Matter, Dark Energy, and the Human Etheric body.'

Guruji further brought another screen from an online library book about the usage of Helium on the respiratory track, which is the main problem in the present Corona Virus treatment .The screen read

Heliox therapy for respiratory obstruction

During normal inspiration, airflow is laminar in the smaller airways such as the terminal bronchioles. Large airways have irregular walls and coupled with the higher velocity results in flow that is less organized and thus turbulent.

In turbulent flow, gas velocity is no longer proportional to the pressure gradient but rather to the square root of the pressure gradient, approximately. This means that if turbulent flow is present, increasing the respiratory rate has a smaller effect on flow rate than with laminar flow. By the same token, increasing respiratory effort causes less increase in flow with turbulent than laminar flow. Flow also becomes less dependent on viscosity and instead is inversely proportional to density; therefore, the denser the gas, the slower the flow. This is where the properties of helium can be utilized to potentially benefit the problems associated with airway obstruction [**5**].

The reduction in airways radius with obstruction causes an increase in airways resistance, as demonstrated using the Hagen-Poiseuille equation. This results in an increased work of breathing with eventual fatigue, hypoxia and hypercapnia. Heliox is a trade name and encompasses a range of medical gases aimed at reducing some of the above phenomena. At

present, two commercially available products exist. These are Heliox21 (21%O_2, 79%He) and Heliox28 (28%O_2, 72%He) and assist because of several factors:

Reduction in respiratory distress. Helium is eight times less dense than oxygen and the clinically available Heliox mixture is three times less dense than air. This reduced density of gas results in a lowering of the Reynolds number and thus a return to laminar flow. By increasing laminar flow, the efficiency of breathing is increased. Even where turbulent flow persists, the work of breathing decreases per unit volume [**6**, 7].

Improved respiratory efficiency. The combination of reduced work of breathing, bulk flow shifting distally and the fact that gas molecules diffuse four times faster through Heliox than through air, combine to enhance alveolar ventilation [**8**]. Heliox has been shown to significantly reduce hypercapnia and normalize pH. It enhances the elimination of CO_2, which diffuses four to five times faster through Heliox than through N_2/O_2 mixtures [**9**]. Also, gas distribution within the lung is improved and thus improves the ventilation/perfusion (V/Q) ratio [**10**].

Enhanced respiratory drug delivery. Heliox enhances respiratory drug delivery by increasing the deposition of nebulized drugs in the distal airways [**11, 12**]. This again can be explained by the improved laminar flow patterns with helium-assisted ventilation and reduction in aerosol impaction in the upper airways, which leads to a more uniform and peripheral deposition [**13**].

Buying valuable time. The above factors all work to provide valuable time for concurrent therapies, such as corticosteroids, to work and thus may reduce the need for escalation of treatment [**14, 15**].

The above benefits of helium-oxygen mixtures in airway obstruction would appear to be considerable. However, the role of helium-oxygen mixtures in all settings remains somewhat controversial. Despite the first clinically successful use of Heliox in 1935, it is still not widely available in acute care facilities. Much of the evidence for its use is anecdotal with a paucity of level 1 data. It is also not a treatment in its own right and should in no way be used as a substitute for other airway obstruction treatment modalities. A Cochrane Database Systemic Review in 2003 analyzed all the randomized controlled trials up to 2002 (six papers, of which only two were high quality and one study dealt solely with pediatrics). They summarized that there was no existing evidence for the use of helium-oxygen mixtures for moderate to severe asthma in the emergency department but that their results should be interpreted with caution, owing to the limited number of studies [**16**].

Guruji said, 'I wish some millions of dollars are spent on the research of this as a cure to corona or any other respiratory track virus.'

Guruji continued, 'unless we are able to find a pathway to release some protons or electrons from the inert gas or find a way for the inert gas vibrations to cross the aetherical space in the body and increase the human atomic vibrations, the cure of diseases and immortality is still some distance away.'

In the present circumstances, the lowest valency and highest vibrating metal that human beings know of is gold. In its purest form, the metal gold has a valency of 1 only and thus has the capability of having maximum vibrations. It is thus the most energetic metal.'

'Therefore, ideally if you eat in gold plates and utensils and cook your food also in utensils made of this metal then it prolongs life. You could also keep gold in its purest form in your bedroom for the same purpose. Now, this is very expensive proposition and therefore not very practical. But, we still recommend that you do the next best thing, which is using silver, which vibrates a shade below gold. Therefore anyone who can afford to do so should adopt silver utensils for cooking and eating to reduce diseases and prolong longer life till a research on the inert gases can give humans the key to immortality. Freeing inert gases of its electrons will create the highest grade of energy on earth and this can lead to immortality or near immortality. And by immortality I do not mean living through your thoughts or ideas, or even taking on another body after having exhausted your feelings in this life. I actually mean living with the body that you have in this present life.'

'The highest energy objects on which research is being done are black holes, which have such high energy levels that they can suck planets into them. The aim of our discussions is to focus on the energy play in the comparatively smaller field of human beings and the influence that it has in propelling life with knowledge. This is especially important after the pandemic as it might provide insights into how to live healthily by discharging your lessons.'

'In conclusion, let's summarize some things that we have learned. We have spoken about the various planes on which we should act to make our life free of bondages and to exhaust all the elements for which this body has taken a birth. We have looked at the various kind of diseases that can afflict the physical body and how to handle them. We have seen how to achieve some wants in this life and improve relationships. We also saw the great message of "love all, serve all" as the simple means of achieving eternal happiness which we shall carry with us as long as we live. The knowledge has been provided for you to assimilate and then act upon, discarding any shade of fear and believing in surrendering yourself to god.'

19

Renunciation and Doubt Clarifications!

Guruji said, 'we are now nearing the end of our conversation today, so I want to talk about the offbeat subject of renunciation. We had touched upon this earlier, and I remember promising you that we would revisit it later in our discussions. So, here is the time when we should do exactly that. When you had come to India last year, Ruth had wanted to go and see some hermits who lived in remote mountain caves. John, if you remember, you had asked me if I could take you to some such hermit who could live in caves, braving the heat and cold, and yet remain blissfully happy. We couldn't go to see some such soul due to bad weather conditions, but let me tell you about them.'

'There are some real people who have renounced the material world as a matter of choice. Let me also warn you that there are some fakes as well. Is renunciation simply to give up modern life? The answer is no. Renunciation is essentially giving up the feelings or impressions of the causal body so

that your unfulfilled thoughts, desires, feelings, or impressions do not compel you to come again to this world. In Hinduism, we believe that once these are exhausted, a person gets into a blissful existence and the enjoyment of life reaches another level. So much so that you automatically tend to be not attached to this world while continuing to live in it. Therefore, whether you are living on a remote mountain or in the heart of Boston is immaterial. In a state of renunciation, non-attachment is both your choice and circumstances. The pleasure of life and health that you will experience is beyond words.'

Guruji folded his hands in a Namaste and said, 'I have given you all that I had for the welfare of mankind. Now, if you have any questions to ask, please do so.'

I asked "Guruji, the knowledge that we have been privileged to get from you is deep and profound. How do we apply it practically? In life, we are all emotional as well as intelligent and these qualities often contradict some of the things that you have recommended that we implement. Managers these days are told to improve their emotional quotients. How do we then implement your recommendations that contradict our emotions?"

Guruji replied, 'Actually, John, there are no contradictions in what I have told you and whatever are you asking. I have told you that whenever you are faced with something, simply apply two criteria – "Love all and serve all". The definition of love, as we discussed, is not what generally you feel as lust but it is a feeling of fellowship with all human beings who have the same energy as you have but are on a different side of the table as per their karma. Emotion is an attachment and

therefore does not let you decide what your correct duty is. So please start differentiating between love and emotions too.'

'Besides, I have also indicated that if you analyze each and every thought that comes to your mind to see whether the thought has come on account of selfishness, greed, lust, or any other cause, then you will be able to distinguish between emotion and rightful duty. If you act according to your duty and without worrying about what conditions or outcome it can produce it will give you self-satisfaction. This self-satisfaction is well worth the effort if you fail, and will give you a rightful place if you succeed.'

'So rightful duty, rather than success or failure, should be a part of your decision-making process.'

Let me tell you one last story. In ancient India, a great war was fought between the ethical and unethical forces that were dominant in those days. This story has been compiled into the Mahabharata, which is one of our epics and also the world's longest epic poem. In this epic, there is a character who was noble, brave, and strong. He is sworn to protect his nation at all times. So, he continues to do so even though the rulers of his nation indulge in practices that are against humanity. He takes part in the great war on the side of the unethical forces of those times. Was his duty to protect his country or its rulers rightful? It clearly wasn't. Anything that harms others and life in general just to pump and maintain our own ego of superiority cannot be considered rightful duty.'

'Similarly, there was another character in this epic who was ethical, but not as strong as the army of the unethical. So, his mental state was to avoid the war because he was worried

that if he loses the battle then his prestige as one of the premier warriors of the time would be shattered. So he started making all kinds of excuses to avoid fighting, simply because of his fear of losing. It is then that the rightful duty is narrated to him by god incarnate, who tells him that you must fight for a right cause and not for fear of the results of that fight. The outcome is that this warrior sheds his self-doubts and fights and wins the war.'

'So rightful duty is acting without promoting ego and without fear. These two are elementary to understand the rightful duty in today's world. So we say that "Help Ever, Hurt Never" is our rightful duty.'

I asked, 'Guruji, sometimes our actions are misinterpreted by others leaving us wondering as to why that was the case. Why does this happen and how should this be handled?'

Guruji replied, 'we have discussed about Karma and that Karmas have to be exhausted as well, irrespective of what you have planned in this life. So we need to remember this knowledge and keep our mind free of any guilt on this account. We have seen that astrologically some relationships will be good, some would result in animosity, and difference of views will persist. We try to correct it by curative astrology to the extent possible but in the end have to take refuge in the knowledge that there are karmas which have to be exhausted and that we are not this body but a bundle of feelings which also has to be exhausted to gain liberation from the cycle of death and life.'

"Guruji, there is so much sorrow in the world and we see some people suffering a lot. What can be done for them?' asked Stella.

Guruji replied, 'It is good to have compassion. So serve them however you can. But, really speaking, there is no sorrow or joy in the world. It is all in how you define the circumstances. Suppose you are rich and are enjoying a good meal, then it would be ok to say that you are joyful. But suppose that you were to receive a call during you meal informing you that all your riches are lost on account of the pandemic, will there be joy left in the wonderful meal, thereafter? So joy was related to those circumstances and knowledge or gyan says don't grieve try to rebuild it with whatever wisdom you have. This is the reason we say "God you are if you feel you are God and dust you are if you feel you are dust". So remember the knowledge which I have imparted to you in all our talks.'

I asked, 'Guruji, is it a sin to have money?'

Guruji laughed and said, 'Who told you this? Nothing is bad or good in life. It is how you use it that could be good or bad. The money or wealth can be used in different ways — you could gamble with it or use it to increase your body comfort. You could donate it to charities or hoard it in banks or gold or whatever. Now, in what circumstance you'd consider your money well-spent depends upon your mind set. Let me tell you another story of a merchant in India who would gamble in the stock market every day. However, he'd spend all that he earned on charity. Therefore he used his skill at gambling to earn for others. So how will you describe his activities? All of us similarly act in this world according to the skills that we have and therefore earn money. But how you use your money finally only defines whether it is sin, ignorance, or praise worthy.'

'The world will continue to have warfare and natural

calamities until a majority of us change our intentions and behavior. Wars are brought about by widespread material selfishness and if we can omit the individual, business, political, national, or even religious selfishness then we will have no wars.'

'Similarly if we are concerned about natural calamities of floods, earthquakes and other disasters we need to see what we as humans are doing? Continuous exploitation of wealth from the ocean disturbs the earth's plates and continuous emissions disturb the ecology and we have more natural disasters.'

'Obviously we cannot completely omit them but don't we think we need to somewhere start to respect nature?'

Stella asked, 'Guruji, we are Christians as you know. We have been given Ten Commandments. How would you explain the commandments to us scientifically?'

Guruji replied, 'Firstly, I think that the Ten Commandments are actually ten rules of happiness. Once you understand the real meaning of the commandments, then happiness will prevail.'

'The first commandment says" thou shalt have no other gods before me." This means that you should have no other priorities before god. However, today our last priority is for god and the first is for the material world. When we give priority to god, we will follow all good practices which we have discussed and happiness will come by itself.'

'The second commandment says, 'Thou shalt not make unto thee any graven image." This means that if you worship the cross of the Christ and forget what the cross stands for then we are worshipping the graven image. We cannot wor-

ship the image and forget what it represents. The words of Jesus saying, "forgive them, my lord, for they know not what they are doing" should be the focal point.'

'The third commandment says 'Thou shalt not take the name of the lord thy god in vain". This means that we cannot just simply chant the name of god without concentration and from the deepest corners of our heart. You could go to church but still be thinking of the material world. Any prayer that you make in that state of mind will be mechanical and in violation of this commandment.'

The fourth commandment says, "Remember the Sabbath day to keep it holy". In Christianity, the Sunday is to keep holy with stillness and self analysis. Sabbath is not a forced duty. It is with joy that we need to enjoy it. But we all know how most people spend their Sundays. So let me not go into the details of that.'

'The fifth commandment says, "Honor thy father and thy mother"

Our parents are representing god's duty when they bring us in this world. Giving them respect, love, and attention is our first duty. In Hinduism, parents are considered the first gods for the child as they are the ones that teach the child and make the child capable of withstanding life and this world.'

The sixth commandment, "Thou shalt not kill," means that you have to control your anger, jealousy, and greed to kill. These are all sermons to exhaust our causal body feeling and impressions.'

'The seventh commandment, "Thou shalt not commit adultery." Do I need to explain this as to why human beings

commit adultery? The emotion or attachment to do adultery should be taken out of our mind.'

The eighth commandment is, "Thou shalt not steal". Many people think that if they steal when no one is looking, then it is ok. But that is not true. Stealing is a habit and you know the emotions behind it. The same needs to be done away with the knowledge that we have acquired now.'

The ninth commandment is "Thou shalt not bear false witness against thy neighbor." The emotions stressed here are reliance on truth on one hand as well as the act of testifying wrongly on account of jealousy or revenge. This needs to be completely done away with. Again we see the omission of feelings or impressions of the causal body.'

The tenth commandment is, "Thou shalt not covet thy neighbor's house, thou shalt not covet thy neighbor's wife, nor his man servant, nor his maid servant, nor his ox, nor his ass, nor any thing that is thy neighbor's." this commandment emphasizes the importance of harmonious living with all human beings. This controls the impressions of the causal plane again.'

Guruji said, 'Now you can see that the purpose of these Ten Commandments was to again exhaust your causal plane feelings or impressions. Control on a mental and causal plane is needed for this.'

'In this world, we know of six types of pleasures though they are only limited to this world. They are healthy body, abundant wealth, vibrant spouse, obeying children, good neighbors, and powerful friends or term it powerful connections with the king.'

The purpose of this life as I have described before is to live

happily, healthily, and to exhaust all impressions and feelings of the causal body. You need to understand the deeper meaning within the Ten Commandments than just focus on the words. You must understand and act on the commandments.'

Guruji paused and smiled benevolently at us. 'Any more questions?' he asked.

I asked, 'Guruji the commandments ask us to not commit adultery. So is it ok to have sexual relations with many partners before marriage?'

Guruji laughed and said, 'Certainly, such relations are less damaging than having multiple extra marital relationships. We have to remember, "Help ever hurt never." So if our action hurts someone then we are not able to exhaust our causal plane feelings or impressions. But this is not to say that sexual relations before marriage, which takes place because of body attraction and for satisfying the ego, are good.'

'However I must also tell you that sexual meditation is another kind of meditation used by some people to exhaust the feelings or impressions. In fact, during the sexual act, a stage of thoughtlessness happens. If this continues for a longer duration without the loss of seminal fluid but simply with the feeling of happiness toward all the organs of the body to let them visually feel happy, it constitutes a meditation practice used by many. You have to absorb the sexual power without losing the seminal fluid and develop great mental powers to write, paint, or express your creativity in a thousand ways. You are essentially spiritualizing the sexual energy as a creative energy and achieving peace, love and bliss in god as well as demonstrating wonderful achievements in the world. And

some day, when you procreate as an objective of the god, then you will really create wonderful citizens of the human kind.'

Guruji looked at his watch and once again bestowed a smile upon us. He was clearly satisfied that he had given us a ton of unknown and known knowledge in a form that was consumable by the entire human community. He had discussed ways that needed to be further researched and also told us about some ayurvedic and herbal treatments, which are not currently permitted in the US though they were available in some other parts of the world. He also appeared satisfied that with the help of astrology and by urging us to know the axis of life, the human energy can get into a better direction. Guruji concluded by saying, 'The pandemic will come and go and you will rebuild whatever has been lost. So live with knowledge after the pandemic. May god bless you all. And remain happy always.'

GLOSSARY

Ashtanga Yoga - The eight necessary habits of human beings which can make them exhaust their past birth feelings or impressions and thus liberate them while allowing happy and healthier life.

Ayurveda - The Indian system of treatment by herbs and some metals singularly or in some combination with each other claiming to eliminate root causes of the disease.

Amla - Known as Gooseberry, is a fruit available in tropical climates and is supposed to rejuvenate the cells.

Asura - Primarily people who have demonic qualities and reside as in habitant of below the earth or hell.

Avatar - A term used in Hinduism as an incarnation of a godly universal energy on the earth to eliminate evils.

Brahma - A universal energy which is also considered as godly energy responsible for the creation of this universe.

Bhakti yoga - A condition in which devotion to the god or universal energy takes place and thus remains happy and healthier.

Deva - Primarily people who have godly qualities and reside as inhabitant of heaven.

Guruji - A knowledgeable person who can advise, guide, and impart wisdom in India known as guruji.

Gyan Yoga - A condition in which supreme knowledge one strives and obtains and thus remains happy and healthier.

Hiranyakashyapu - A demon king in Hinduism who was so

powerful that godly energy had to destroy him with an unparalleled anger.

Haritaki - A herb used in Indian ayurveda system as a laxative to remove constipation.

Hirak bhasma - An Ayurvedic and astrological medicine prepared by oxidating the fine cuttings essentially carbon obtained during diamond polishing in a micro powdered form given as one of the rejuvenating medicines in India.

Indra - King of heaven and devas or godly persons according to Hinduism who is powerful but is in constant threat from demons.

Jalandhar Bandh - A breathing exercise where deep breath is taken and chin is brought down to touch the throat thus locking the breath inside and holding it for a while as one of exercise of Pranayama.

Kauravas-one of the cousin groups in the epic war of two cousin kings who were considered to be on the wrong side of the universal energy due to jealousy.

Kapal Bhati - A breathing exercise of pranayama where in the lower abdomen below the navel is pushed inside developing an exhaust of breath out of lungs and nostrils thus cleaning air passage and allowing temperature to flow within the spine freely.

Kapha - A fat or oily mucous or calcium compounds which remain in the body and are not normally excreted and cause diseases.

Laxmi - A goddess of wealth in Hinduism and wife of godly energy Vishnu which is the energy for preservation and born out of drilling ocean in ancient times.

Mahabali - an ancient king who was demonic full of greed but charitable.

Mahesh - A universal fire energy considered as godly in Hinduism for destruction.

Manu - An equivalent of Adam in creation of the life in world.

Mount Kailash - A mountain in Himalayas considered in Hinduism as an abode of one of their eternal gods Shiva and considered holy.

Narsimha - A godly universal energy which came onto earth in form of half lion and half man to destroy demon king Hiranyakashyapu.

OM - A sound which we can create lyrically as OHHHM and which is the first universal energy for creation and is used in some meditation technique also.

Ojas - A condition in which a healthy temperature flow in body is maintained.

Pandavas - Another cousin group in war of two cousin kings, these were on the side of universal energy who fought for the right.

Pitta - A condition described in ayurveda of enzymes and acid secretion in the body to consume food and an excess of which could be a cause of acidic PH blood.

Pranayama - A type of breathing exercise basically to pump in more oxygen in the body by deeper inhalations and exhalations and is combined with Yoga to keep body healthier.

Prahlad - In Hinduism considered son of demon king Hiranyakashyapu and considered having godly qualities and on whose prayers Narsimha appeared and killed the demon king.

Prakriti - The female part of Mother Nature energy and law.

Purusha - The male part of Mother Nature energy and law and the ultimate energy source.

Punarnava - An Ayurvedic herbal drug known as Brahavia

diffusa and is taken for treatment of liver primarily according to the ayurveda system.

Rishi - An Indian scientist in old ancient India who also meditated a lot.

Saptrishis - The original seven inert gases created in the universe.

Shatrupa - An equivalent of Eve in Hinduism responsible as female counterpart to create life.

Shiva - A Hindu godly energy which resides in Mount Kailash in Himalayas.

Shrimad Bhagwatam - A holy book in Hinduism written by great Indian rishi which vide stories of different godly appearance imparts knowledge and reinforces meaning of love and sacrifice.

Shringa Bhasma - An Ayurvedic preparation of oxidizing deer horn and is considered an immunity booster.

Unani - A system of treatment which originated in Greece but now is practiced also in India.

Vaikuntha - In mid of ocean abode of God Vishnu or the universal energy of preservation and the ultimate place of peace.

Vishnu - A universal energy of preservation and considered as light and in Hinduism known as god and husband of Laxmi which is goddess of wealth and thus they preserve human beings.

Varaha - An avatar of energy appearing in the form of boar which helped the land mass of earth come out of water filled in the beginning of creation and thus helped life establishing on earth.

Vata - A condition described in Ayurveda of current flow or blood flow and any obstruction gets converted into disease.

Yaksha - A demi god in Hinduism which is equivalent to angels and is knowledgeable and helpful.

AF539193